PAEDIATRIC NURSING PROCEDURES

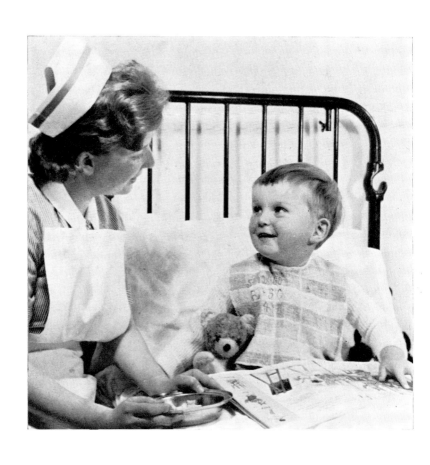

PAEDIATRIC NURSING PROCEDURES

R. M. SACHARIN
R.S.C.N., R.G.N., S.C.M.

Former Assistant Tutor, Royal Hospital for Sick Children, Glasgow;
Former Examiner for the General Nursing Council, Scotland

M. H. S. HUNTER
R.G.N., R.S.C.N., S.C.M., R.C.I.Edin.

Matron, Royal Hospital for Sick Children, Edinburgh;
Examiner for the General Nursing Council, Scotland

Foreword by
RUTH CLARKSON
R.S.C.N., R.G.N.

Formerly Matron, Royal Hospital for Sick Children, Glasgow

SECOND EDITION

E. & S. LIVINGSTONE LTD
EDINBURGH AND LONDON

1969

E. & S. Livingstone Limited 1969

First Edition 1964
Second Edition 1969

SBN 443 00609 1

Printed in Great Britain

FOREWORD

THE tendency of the present age towards specialisation in all fields of Nursing creates a need for books such as this.

It is my privilege in the foreword to pay tribute to the care, time, and attention to detail which the authors have devoted to its production.

I am sure it will find a welcome on the bookshelves of the many whose special interest lies in the nursing of children, and in the training of the paediatric Nurse.

RUTH CLARKSON

1964

PREFACE TO THE SECOND EDITION

WE have been greatly encouraged and pleased by the response to the first edition. The second edition has been brought up to date and many additions have been made. We are again indebted to our colleagues, both nursing and medical, for the help they so willingly gave in the extensive revision of the text.

Chapter I, The Child in Hospital, has been revised and The Importance of Play in Hospital added. The chapter on Ward Infection has been rewritten and brought up to date. A new chapter on Observing the Child and Recording of Vital Signs has been included. The Care of the Premature Infant has been rewritten and additions made to the chapter on Feeding Problems in the Surgical Ward. Techniques and procedures occurring with increasing frequency have been included such as: Peritoneal Dialysis; Renal Biopsy; The Care of the Child with Nasotracheal intubation and Positive Pressure Ventilation. The chapter on Resuscitative Measures has been completely revised. Particular thanks are due to Dr D. J. Grubb, Edinburgh, for constructive help with chapters XII and XX.

We are indebted to Mrs Hamilton, Edinburgh, for her help and patience in typing many of the manuscripts and to Mrs R. A. Hunter for many additional line drawings.

We should also like to thank Messrs E. and S. Livingstone for their co-operation and advice.

R. M. SACHARIN

M. H. S. HUNTER

1969

PREFACE TO THE FIRST EDITION

THE nursing of the sick child demands great skill and understanding which cannot be readily obtained in any short course. We hope that this book will provide some of the answers which the student nurse requires when preparing or actually carrying out the procedure and give an understanding of the child's needs before, during and after any such procedure. The book is intended for student nurses training for the Sick Children's Register, but it is hoped that the student nurse seconded to a Children's Hospital or nursing sick children in a general hospital, will find the book valuable and helpful. In this book the term 'nurse' includes both male and female members of the nursing profession. We have, however, used the feminine gender throughout for the sake of uniformity and simplicity.

We have endeavoured to cover as large a field as possible. New methods of treatment, new equipment and new ideas create a challenge for the student nurse and the trained nurse. To keep abreast of the new discoveries in the medical world, the nurse must be willing to adapt her experience and widen her outlook.

To ensure that procedures are carried out correctly, it is vital that the nurse at all stages of her career should seek to understand the purpose of each procedure. We have given the reason for all procedures and mentioned the diseases where the procedure or treatment may be required. We hope thereby, to stimulate the interest of the nurse to seek further knowledge.

We must emphasise that methods vary widely from hospital to hospital and even from ward to ward in each hospital. Certain procedures, therefore, will have to be adopted to suit the given circumstances and conditions.

We are indebted to the ward sisters, our colleagues, who have helped and encouraged us, to the doctors, nurse tutors and ward sisters who have read the manuscripts and given us their criticisms and advice. They range from the north of Scotland to the south of England. We are grateful for the contributions of Miss Wardlaw, formerly orthopaedic ward sister and Miss Sutherland, M.D., F.R.S.C.E. for her chapter on Feeding Problems in the Surgical

Child; to Miss Henderson for her chapter on Physiotherapy and also to Dr S. P. Rawson for his guidance in the chapter on Radiological procedures. We are also indebted to Miss Cleary and Mrs M. Benjamin of Glasgow, and Mrs Jackson of Edinburgh for their help and patience in typing many of the manuscripts; to Mr Devlin of the Royal Hospital for Sick Children, Glasgow, and Miss Brydone of the Royal Hospital for Sick Children, Edinburgh, for the excellent photographs. The line drawings are the work of Mrs R. A. Hunter. Their clarity speak for themselves and we are grateful for all the time she has spent on them. We should also like to thank Mr C. Macmillan, and Mr J. Parker of Messrs E. and S. Livingstone, Publishers, for their cooperation and advice and Miss L. McDonald, M.A., B.A. for her critical reading of the manuscript and valuable suggestions.

                                                    R. M. SACHARIN
1964   M. H. S. HUNTER

LIST OF CONTENTS

CHAPTER I

THE CHILD IN HOSPITAL

CHILDREN in hospital present difficult and complex problems. Each child with his own personality in the developing stage, each with varying habits and behaviour, provides for the nurse a challenging situation. Only intelligent understanding of the needs of each child will help the nurse in her relationship with him.

It is important to remember that the child has suddenly been uprooted and placed into an environment which is both strange and frightening to him. The fact that he is an ill child and has to receive treatment of some kind will increase his fear and anxiety.

If the child shows obvious signs of illness, it is comparatively easy for the nurse to be compassionate. Often the child is weak and completely dependent on the nurse. Greater difficulty is experienced with the active child who may be resentful and frightened or timid and withdrawn. In both cases fear is the motivating force, fear of the unknown, strange surroundings, uniforms, strange people, or, in many cases, fear of a falsely presented picture of hospital life.

Preparation for hospitalisation would help the child to form a picture of what might be expected. This of course will depend on the age of the child. Up to the age of four, it is not advisable for the mother to go into any great detail about what is going to happen, but the child must be told that he is going into hospital. It should be explained to him that his mother will not be able to stay with him, except in those hospitals which have a mother and child unit. He should be reassured that his parents will visit him as often as it is possible. Older children will ask questions and will require a more detailed explanation, but again it is dependent on the child himself how much he can be told. Hospital authorities can also help by issuing booklets giving information and showing pictures of hospital life. If the child is for elective admission, there is greater opportunity for preparing him. It will be of help if the child could visit the ward, meet the sister and

B

nurses who will be looking after him and see the other children. The first impression is of vital importance. The waiting room should have toys which the child can play with while awaiting admission. The nurse should acquaint herself with the child's name before introducing herself, so that he feels already expected. She should sit with the mother and child and make them feel at ease by talking to them for a short while, before beginning the admission procedure. Where possible, the mother should be encouraged to undress, even bath the child, and see him settled in bed.

Before leaving the ward, the parents should be given an opportunity to discuss with a senior member of the ward nursing team any problem or specific personal details relating to their child. This would give them the impression that a personal interest is taken and makes parting from their child easier.

If the mother has brought the child's own toys, or any object, such as a piece of blanket, to which he is very attached and which gives him a sense of comfort, these should be left with him or be readily available. The child's locker should be so placed and designed that he has easy access to it.

Questions such as 'When will my mummy be coming?' should be answered honestly. For the 3-5 year old, the time factor has no meaning. A specific time, e.g. after dinner or teatime, can be mentioned if the approximate time of the parent's visit is known.

The ideal situation for the child under five who has to be admitted to hospital would be to have his mother with him to share his hospitalisation (as is done in some hospitals). This prevents emotional trauma and helps to hasten his recovery. Where this is not possible free visiting hours can do much to maintain the mother-child relationship.

For the older child, regular visiting helps to maintain the close family bond and relieve some of the tension and anxiety which is often associated with hospitalisation. During these visiting periods the parents should be encouraged to take an active part in the nursing of their child; e.g. help with the feeding, playing, reading to him, and tucking him up for the night.

The Infant

This age-group probably presents the least problems to the nurse. Normally the infant feeds and sleeps, but it is often forgotten that physical contact is essential to the infant to avoid emotional starvation. Infants must be spoken to and held lovingly. It is not just enough to feed and change the child and put him into his cot. The nurse should also play and talk with him to evoke response in the infant. When parents visit their infants, the mother should be allowed to nurse her infant whenever possible. Visiting could be arranged so that it coincides with the feeding of the infant. As nurses, we are apt to forget not only the infant's but also the mother's needs and we must be willing to return to the mother her function as mother, at every available opportunity.

The Pre-school Child

This age-group is by far the most difficult to handle in hospital. Children vary in their ability to speak, which is often associated with the social and economic background in which the child grows up. It also depends on his status in the family and on his stage and rate of development. It is often difficult to make out or understand his wants; it is therefore essential to find out from his parents as much as possible about his speaking habits; for example, special words for his toilet requirements. It is also important to ascertain which 'milestones' have been achieved; for example, feeding, speaking, toilet training, thus ensuring too much is not expected of the child.

Food fads and tantrums are very common and must be dealt with as they arise. Food should be made as interesting as possible. Small portions are given at first, which can be repeated if desired. Where a large number of children sit at a table with a nurse supervising, little difficulty is experienced during meal times. The greatest difficulty is with the child who is confined to bed. Reading a story will help to overcome this difficult episode. The small child can be lifted on to the nurse's knees, and where possible, the child should be allowed to feed himself or help to do so. At all events, scenes should be avoided and a calm atmosphere maintained. When tantrums occur, it is probably best to allow the child to get over them. It is important not to make him feel 'bad', but to make him realise that his difficulties are understood. Reassurance should be given as soon as the tantrum is over. A certain amount of regression is considered normal. Independence should be encouraged or re-established where regression has taken place; e.g. in feeding and dressing himself.

Constipation is common for some days after admission. Here it is advisable to enlist the help of the mother in re-establishing normal bowel habits, rather than treating the constipation with aperients. Bedwetting and soiling often occur in children of this age-group while in hospital and must be regarded as symptoms of anxiety. The child should never be scolded but every effort made to reassure him. Where the child has already been toilet trained at home, it is important that frequent opportunities should be given to the child to use the potty. Where possible, a special nurse should be assigned to supervise this important function. During visiting time, mothers could be of enormous help here. If the child has not been toilet trained and is going to be in hospital for a short while, it is not wise to attempt it, because in a strange and frightening environment it will lead to frustration and is rarely successful. This does not apply to children who have to remain in hospital for a long time. Here it is important that 'potting' of the children should become part of the day's routine.

When treatment has to be carried out, the nurse should explain very simply what she is going to do. Reasoning is difficult, particularly if the child is in a state of terror. She should, therefore, calm the child and impress upon him that she wants to help him to get better. It is never wise to carry out a procedure on an unsuspecting child. The nurse has the greatest opportunity to recognise the needs of the apprehensive child. She should notify the doctor accordingly, so that adequate sedation can be given beforehand.

Importance of Play to the Child

For a young child play is of the utmost importance. It is not merely a means of passing the time but plays a vital part in helping him to come to terms with his environment and to help him deal with the strains and stresses of daily living. Experience gained through play will be assimilated thereby helping him to adapt to new situations.

When the child is admitted to hospital his security is disturbed and even where there is a relatively happy atmosphere it is likely to be a traumatic experience. It is therefore understandable that play is often of a destructive kind and may well reflect the child's anger and show his inability to cope with the situation. The small child in particular is often enclosed in a small space and left to his own devices for long periods. He has difficulty in communicating his fears and anxieties and either cries for his mother and lies or sits quietly, giving the impression of having 'settled down'. In fact this behaviour is one that requires urgent attention to prevent serious emotional trauma. Where and when possible the child should be lifted up, cuddled and talked to.

In a busy ward where the number of nurses is inadequate it is extremely difficult to find time for playing with or giving the child an opportunity to play effectively. It would, therefore, be ideal if an adult trained in nursery school work could be part of the ward team. This would not only provide the child with someone who would read to him or guide him in his play, but would also be a stable figure in a ward where constant changes of staff have a very disturbing effect on him.

Before one can consider what kind of play to initiate it is essential to recognise that all children differ in their rate of development. It might help therefore to give some guidance on the type of toys suitable for different age-groups.

The Small Infant

After birth the infant spends most of the time sleeping. Gradually, the sleeping period decreases and as he grows older he becomes more capable of receiving and reacting to external impressions. His early discoveries concern mainly himself and his earliest play activities are concerned with movement. For example, he will lie and kick, play with his fingers and toes and stretch his limbs. Gradually he will learn to manipulate toys and pick up those which are near him. He will soon reach the stage when he likes to put on and take off, take out and put back objects. A great deal of repetition is the general pattern of play.

Type of Toys. Toys must be easy to hold, therefore the material must be light. They should be unbreakable and non-inflammable, washable and colours must be fast. Soft toys must be manufactured under hygienic conditions and only good materials used. It is also important to ensure that the toys do not contain any dangerous parts.

By the end of the first year most babies are able to crawl, shuffle, stand or walk. Pushing and pulling toys are very useful. These should be strongly constructed and well balanced.

One to Two Years Old

This is the toddler stage when children attempt to climb, so extra care is required. At the same time, he should be allowed to climb and explore provided it is safe to do so. For those children who are confined to bed it is likely to be a frustrating time and they are often restless and impatient. While they are confined to bed, toys, such as interlocking cubes, building beakers and pegs are useful. Drawing with crayons is enjoyed, but the bed would have to be protected. Picture books are important and here the nurse can use mealtimes to read to him while feeding him. At this stage children play on their own, but require constant supervision. They are inquisitive and will play with anything within their reach and great care must be taken so that small objects, such as beads, are kept out of their reach.

Two to Three Years Old

Play becomes more organised. His manipulative skills are improving and he is able to assemble quite complicated toys.

They will enjoy playing with wooden trains with interlocking carriages, building bricks, simple jig-saws, pencil and paper, hammering pegs. Picture books and very short stories, nursery rhymes and singing are very important. While in bed he can be given a large box or tin in which he can store any oddment that takes his fancy. At this stage the child has periods when he likes adults to play with him, but generally he is quite happy to play on his own near adults or other children.

Three to Four Years Old

This is the stage of imitation. They like to join in the activities of the adult. While at home, the child will help with cleaning, dusting and cooking. This is not possible in hospital, particularly when he is confined to bed. Imitation can still take place by allowing the child to play at nurses and doctors with their dollies. This helps them to act out some of the anxieties which hospital life generates. When he is allowed up he should be given every opportunity to play adequately. Singing and story telling are very important and can be organised whether they are confined to bed or allowed up.

This age-group use a greater variety of toys, some of which include: doll and doll's clothing, ironing board and iron, trains, cars, jigsaws, paper and pencils (coloured), bead threading, picture sewing, water and sand.

FOUR TO FIVE YEARS OLD

Great changes have taken place since babyhood. He is now a capable child, probably able to dress and feed himself. He is able to speak and has generally no difficulty in making himself understood, though there are children who have difficulty in so doing. He is generally constructive in his play but destructive play still occurs. He is now able to create situations and events and shows imagination in his play. When playing with others, it will now become something definite, like a house, train, etc. He will spend longer periods at one game as his powers of concentration increase. This is also the stage when the companionship of other children will be sought. Drawing plays an important part and the child must be allowed to experiment both with shapes and colours. Gradually the drawing or painting will show a definite theme. It may not be clear to the adult, but it is very clear to the child because in it he is expressing his inner thoughts and feelings. Children should be left to do the drawings themselves and help should only be given when the child asks for it.

Cutting out is enjoyed greatly but will require supervision, particularly when he is confined to bed. Special nursery scissors are available which are small, light and have a rounded point. Making objects from clay or Plasticine gives a great deal of satisfaction. The bed would need to be protected. Any other previously mentioned toys are also used by this age-group, but the play will vary with the maturity of the individual child. Stories are very important and short story sessions should be held whenever possible.

The School Child

This age-group shows varying degrees of understanding, and explanations can be given which are more readily accepted. These children are usually co-operative and are more apt to give the impression of being brave, yet the nurse should realise that behind this façade lies fear of the unknown. The child should be encouraged to talk about his fears and worries. These could retard improvement of his condition. Guidance can be given in the choice of books and a supply of books and toys should be available for all age-groups. It is also important to remember that the older child is eager to know about his illness and progress, and care must be taken to ensure that he does not inadvertently overhear discussions about his own or any other child's condition. Verbal reports should not be given at his bedside or in his hearing, but it is equally important that the child should be told of any progress he is making towards recovery.

Where nursing procedures are carried out, nurses should realise that they are caring for human beings who, though small, have a well-defined sense of shame and a need for privacy. This need must be respected and screens provided when treatment is being given or bedpans issued outwith the normal bedpan periods. Where the child performs his own toilet, he should be given the opportunity to wash his hands. When examinations are carried out necessitating undressing, the nurse should cover the child with a light blanket and not expose him to the view of onlookers.

If he is well enough, a few hours of schoolwork will keep him abreast with the school curriculum and close co-operation between teacher and nursing staff is essential. The teacher should be encouraged to discuss difficulties which may be due to the child's illness or some underlying worry both about his condition and his schoolwork.

The maintenance of discipline presents some difficulty which is often aggravated by lack of occupation. This could be overcome by ensuring that the children are occupied with some form of constructional activity. This may require supervision, particularly where handwork of some kind is involved. It would not only give them something to do but also create interest and a sense of achievement. Some examples of the kind of work older children can do include:

For girls—sewing, embroidery, knitting, drawing and painting.

For boys—simple building sets, Meccano sets, weaving, mat making, drawing and painting.

Although children may be confined to bed, where possible they should be allowed to move and play about. Firmness is essential but it is not advisable to apply too many restrictions. Older children who are allowed up should be encouraged to help by playing with younger children and helping with their meals.

It will be appreciated that reactions to situations vary with each individual, with age and with the type and extent of the illness. The nurse should learn to evaluate the child's reaction and behaviour and respond to it with patience, understanding and love.

This will help to minimise the psychological trauma which the hospital experience can produce.

The Nurse and the Parents

Parents' reactions vary greatly when their children are admitted to hospital. This depends partly on the reason for the admission. Some are openly aggressive towards the nursing staff while others are co-operative in every way. As nurses we must understand the dilemma in which the parents find themselves. They may feel guilty at the state of ill health of their child in which case they are probably afraid of criticism, and the natural reaction is that of aggressive behaviour. On the other hand, they may resent handing over their child to someone else (in this case the nurse) who, they feel will take their place and also may win the child's affection. This will be resented and in their resentment they will probably find faults in the nursing of the child.

The problem is how to approach the more difficult parents. As already mentioned, first impressions play a very important part. When receiving the parents at the ward door, it is important to remember that the nurse is a hostess welcoming her visitors. Officiousness and abruptness must never be permitted at any time. Often this behaviour of the nurse is part of a desire to impress, but the parents will be much more impressed if they are approached by a well-mannered, kindly nurse.

When parents are visiting their children, the nurse in charge should be available to answer any question which they may have. All relevant information should be ascertained beforehand from the doctor and/or sister, so that as many questions as possible may be answered freely and without hesitation. A visitor's book should be kept indicating that the child has been visited and that information has been given regarding the child's progress. When talking to the parents the nurse should not talk down to them but talk in a friendly way. She should remember that all her statements must be clear and concise. Personal opinions about the child's disease should not be given but questions involving the child's eating and sleeping progress may be asked, and should be answered honestly.

While visiting their child, parents may be aware that changes in his behaviour or personality have been or are taking place. This can cause real distress. The cause, if known, should be explained to them; e.g. Cortisone can produce marked changes both in his physical appearance as well as in his behaviour. A child who previously was happy and contented may become irritable and selfish. This may well be an unconscious desire to punish his parents and will require a great deal of patience and understanding. It does not mean that the parents should become over-indulgent, but firmness should be tempered with love and understanding. Many parents feel that every visit to their child must include a present of some kind. It should be explained to them that this is neither necessary nor desirable. The visiting period should be used as a modified extension of home-life. The parents can play games with or read stories to their children or just be there. Another problem which presents itself is the child who has had frequent and often long periods in an acute hospital. Unless there is support and co-operation from the parents such children could present disciplinary problems.

When the mother appears to be over-anxious, it is of great value to find out the cause of her worries and give her the opportunity to talk about them. Here, the nurse must be a good and sympathetic listener. A mother who feels that she is treated with sympathy and understanding will eventually also be more co-operative. This in turn will make her feel easier at leaving her child in hospital.

Extended visiting periods mean that student nurses at different levels of training may be consulted by the parents, when they are temporarily left in charge of the ward. This may frighten the young nurse, who may have the desire to hide herself rather than face a barrage of questions which she feels unable to answer. Alternatively a nurse finding herself in such a situation may herself behave in an aggressive manner in an effort to overcome her inability to cope with the situation. The young nurse must learn to face this difficult situation. Guidance and instruction should be given on the approach to the parents and a full report given to the nurse before she is left to cope with this responsibility. It should be impressed upon the nurse that any questions put to her are not meant to be an examination of her knowledge but express a desire of the parents to obtain information regarding their child's condition and progress. Where any doubt exists as to what to tell the parents, she can ask them kindly to await the return of sister or the charge nurse.

Telephone enquiries bring their own problems. Misunderstandings often occur and to avoid this happening simply phrased sentences are used in reply. These replies could be informative without going into detail about specific treatments given. The standard reply of 'he has had a good day or night' could surely be made more informative; e.g. 'John has slept well all night and he is bright and happy' if that is the case, or 'John is taking his feeds or meals eagerly', or otherwise. It is important that the nurse should mention the child's christian name. This makes it much more personal and also gives the enquirer the impression that the nurse knows about whom she is in fact reporting.

Every parent should be given the opportunity to speak to the doctor in charge of the ward. When the interview is taking place, the sister or nurse in charge should always be present. Parents often feel in awe of the doctor and are over-anxious, therefore they may be unable to comprehend what is said to them. This often means that the nurse has to repeat and translate in simple yet correct language what the doctor has said to them.

Children without Visitors

A great number of children who are in hospital may be without visitors either for long periods or throughout their stay in hospital. It is important that records should be kept indicating whether each child has been visited. The hospital medical social worker plays an important part here by acting as liaison between parents and hospital, and should, therefore, be contacted to determine the reason for the absence of the parents. The importance of visiting should be stressed and any necessary help provided. This liaison will elicit information about the child's home environment which may help in the final decision when to discharge the child from hospital.

The nurse should endeavour to find opportunities to play with such children giving them extra attention particularly during the visiting period. Parents of other children are very helpful and understanding and it will be found that they readily visit these children. On the other hand it will be found that a child who is allowed up will attach himself to another child's mother, who will often respond. This situation, although not ideal, appears to satisfy most children and fill in a lonely part of their day. For the child who has to remain in hospital for a long period, it will be necessary to find a person, preferably a relative or someone known to the child, who can act as mother substitute and visit him frequently.

BIBLIOGRAPHY

Benz, G. (1964). *Paediatric Nursing.* St. Louis: Mosby.
Bowley, A. H. (1961). *The Psychological Care of the Child in Hospital.* Edinburgh: Livingstone.
Haller, J. A. (1967). *The Hospitalised Child and his Family.* London: Oxford University Press.
Illingworth, R. S. (1967). *The Development of the Infant and Young Child*, 3rd ed. Edinburgh: Livingstone.
Illingworth, R. S. (1968). *The Normal Child*, 4th ed. London: Churchill.
Marlow, D. (1965). *Textbook of Paediatric Nursing*, 2nd ed., Chaps. 3 & 4. Philadelphia: Saunders.
Ministry of Health (1959). *The Welfare of Children in Hospital.* London: H.M.S.O.
Noble, E. (1967). *Play and the Sick Child.* London: Faber & Faber.

CHAPTER II

OBSERVING AND RECORDING

Observing; recording temperature, pulse, respiration and blood pressure; vital signs of children with head injury; vital signs of children with convulsions; fluid and electrolyte balance.

OBSERVING

THE art of nursing the sick child lies not merely in carrying out procedures efficiently but depends primarily on the ability of the nurse to observe the child effectively and report accurately any deviation from the accepted norm. The nurse has many opportunities in observing the child and her reports will be of great value to the doctor.

The child's physical and emotional response to illness can be so unlike that of adults that those inexperienced in the care of the child may fail to observe clues of critical importance. In general, the child responds in a more dramatic way. There may be little time from the first early warning sign to the development of a serious situation.

The small child has little or no means of communicating his difficulties or pain and it is here that his mother has a vital part to play. She knows his normal behaviour and response, and her comments and observations must always be sought. There is the added problem that the child's symptoms can be masked by the distress of admission to hospital. It is, therefore, of the utmost importance that the nurse learns how to gain the confidence and trust of the child.

Observation of the child includes recognition of the abnormal or the unusual, be this in behaviour or in physical manifestations. A knowledge of normal physiology is essential if abnormalities in body functions are to be recognised. The physical and mental development of the child at any age has been the subject of detailed studies and average standards have been calculated which help to assess a child's attainments. Children differ in their rate of growth and development so that variations of attainment can still be within the accepted range. The growth of a child (physical, intellectual and emotional) is dependent upon his innate potentialities and the environmental factors surrounding him. It is not our aim to go into details about the norm or milestones attainable at different age levels, but rather to mention some important aspects to be observed and recorded when caring for the sick child.

The following questions will be of assistance in obtaining a general assessment of the child:

1. DEVELOPMENTAL ATTAINMENTS
   What developmental attainments should the child have reached for his age and how does his present condition compare with these?
2. RESPONSE TO NEW SITUATIONS
   (*a*) Is the child too ill to show much response?
   (*b*) Does he appear very dependent on his mother, or is he able to relinquish some of his dependency? This will vary with the age and emotional growth of the child.
   (*c*) What is the mother's response to the new situation? Her reactions will provide a link in understanding the child's attitudes and behaviour.
3. THE HISTORY AND DIAGNOSIS OF THE CONDITION
   What special signs and symptoms should be looked for?

In effect, the nurse requires to make a comparative study of the child and to use this knowledge when she makes each assessment.

GENERAL OBSERVATIONS

Crying

The infant uses crying as a means of expressing himself; it is also a means of exercising his lungs.

1. Anger or rage. He will scream, kick and may hold his breath for a few seconds. This is his way of letting us know his needs. Hunger can produce an angry cry.

2. Pain. When the infant is in pain, he utters a shrill or piercing sound and may give some indication where the pain lies. For example, if he has colic, he draws up his legs. With earache, there may be constant movement of the head. In meningitis, or cerebral irritation from other causes, a high-pitched scream can be heard.

The attempt to coax a smile which results in an irritable cry is a sure sign that a baby is unwell.

Sleep

Normally, sleep should be deep and restful. Any restlessness or crying out should be noted.

Position

Children normally seldom lie still for very long. Certain positions may be adopted, which should be noted, such as:
1. Lying with the knees drawn up. This is the position of most comfort when there is abdominal pain.
2. Lying face downwards, or burying the face in the bedclothes, as in photophobia.
3. Head retraction with disinclination to move the head is apparent in meningitis.

Behaviour

Behaviour can be indicative not only of emotional disturbances, but also of some physical illness.

Excitement and restlessness occur with hypoglycaemia, while increasing dullness or sleepiness may indicate hyperglycaemia.

Vomiting

This is a common symptom exhibited by the sick child. Important factors to consider are the age of the child in relation to his diet and his manner of feeding or eating. The amount, frequency and character of the vomiting should also be noted.

1. TYPE OF VOMITING
   (a) Effortless, as in the ruminating infant or infant with hiatus hernia.
   (b) Effortless but accompanied with cyanosis or spluttering, as in congenital abnormalities of the gastro-intestinal tract.
   (c) Possetting or vomiting of mouthfuls, mainly found in breast-fed infants and believed to be due to air swallowing.
   (d) Projectile, as in congenital pyloric stenosis.

2. CONTENT
   (a) Food.
   (b) Coffee ground (blood), as in gastric or duodenal ulcers and hiatus hernia.
   (c) Bile, as in intestinal obstruction.
   (d) Mucus, as in vomiting in the new-born infant or in gastro-enteritis.

3. RELATION OF VOMITING to intake of food; e.g. immediately after intake or some time after.

4. AMOUNT AND FREQUENCY: mouthfuls, part of feed, or whole feed. Relationship of the amount vomited to the amount of food or fluid taken.

Sweating

This is an important factor when there is need to maintain an accurate fluid and electrolyte balance. Excessive sweating must, therefore, be reported.

Cough

This is a common symptom in the sick child. Accurate reporting of the type of cough, when it occurs, whether associated with feeding or eating, and the frequency is important.

1. Noisy barking cough, as in laryngeal stridor, occurring usually during the night.
2. Harsh cough associated with pain, as in tracheitis.
3. Spasms of coughing; occurring in bronchitis, bronchiolitis, lipoid pneumonia.
4. Moist, productive cough, as in bronchitis and pneumonia.
5. Unproductive barking cough, as in sino-bronchitis.
6. Paroxysmal type of cough followed by a whoop occurring in whooping cough.

Stools

Observation and reporting of stools are of importance not only to aid diagnosis and treatment but also to assess progress in some diseases. Every unit has its own specific symbols to indicate the type of stool passed. The fact that a stool has been passed must be marked on the appropriate chart.

Any difficulty experienced during defaecation must be reported. Some children may have difficulties using bedpans and it may be necessary, where possible, to allow them up to the toilet. Others will be used to having somebody beside them; this will require patience and readjustment.

The first few stools of a newborn infant are soft in consistency and dark green in colour. They consist of epithelial cells, mucus and bile and are called meconium. Gradually the stool becomes pale yellow and more solid in consistency. The number of stools passed are usually four to five per day for the first few weeks and decrease gradually to one or two per day. There are individual variations with regard to the frequency and also the type passed. Some infants and children may not defaecate daily but provided the stools are normal in colour and consistency and there is no difficulty during the process, then it can be considered as normal.

The detection of abnormal stools is an important responsibility; these can be classified as follows:

1. CONSISTENCY: Whether loose and watery, well formed or as lumps.

2. FREQUENCY: The number of stools passed and the time of greatest frequency.

3. AMOUNT: If loose, the amount may vary—sometimes only a stain; at other times copious soiling may occur. This is important when assessing fluid and electrolyte balance.

4. COLOUR:
   (a) Dark green mucous, as in meconium.
   (b) Green with mucus or blood, as in gastro-enteritis.
   (c) Pale grey and bulky, as in coeliac disease.
   (d) Frothy yellow, as in excessive carbohydrate intake.
   (e) Black may be due to blood or iron intake.
   (f) Small brown mucous, as in chronic ulcerative colitis.

5. ODOUR:
   (a) Sour, as in gastro-enteritis.
   (b) Offensive, as in fibrocystic disease of the pancreas and coeliac disease.

Other abnormal constituents :

   (a) Fat, as in coeliac disease or excessive fat intake.
   (b) Undigested.

(c) Mucus: Slimy appearance, as in enteric infection.
     Mucoid and purulent, as in staphylococcal entero-
     colitis.

(d) Blood: Mixed with mucus, as in dysentery.
     'Redcurrant jelly' (blood and mucus), as in intus-
     susception.

(e) Foreign bodies: worms (threadworms, tapeworms and their
     ova), pips, coins etc.

(f) Drugs: certain drugs change the character of the stools;
     e.g. iron and bismuth produce black stools. Carmine
     marker will give a pink colour.

Urine

See Chapter XIV on urine testing.

RECORDING OF TEMPERATURE

A child's heat regulating mechanism is not fully developed until
the age of 3-4 years. He can, therefore, suddenly become hyperpyrexic or hypothermic. In the initial stages of illness, it is likely
that the temperature should be taken at 4-hourly intervals. In
the gravely ill infant, monitoring equipment may be used in
preference to disturbing the infant by frequent recordings.

A clinical thermometer with a short bulb normally used for
recording the temperature in the rectum is the safest type for use
with a child. The bulb is shorter and thicker and therefore less
likely to break or penetrate rectal tissue.

REQUIREMENTS:

1. Thermometer (container of disinfectant if necessary).
2. Cotton wool in a container.
3. Receptacle for soiled wool.
4. Book for recording temperature, pulse and respirations.

METHOD. To record a skin temperature the thermometer is
shaken to below 35°C or 95°F. The skin is dried in the axilla or
the groin of the younger child, and the thermometer is inserted.
The bulb must be between two skin surfaces and held there
firmly for the time which is stated on the thermometer. The
thermometer is read and the temperature recorded. The bulb
must not be held between the fingers when reading the thermometer.

Since exercise or excessive activity may increase temperature, it is important that the child who is not confined to bed should be at rest for some time before the thermometer is inserted. If the groin is used, care must be taken to remove all traces of talcum powder or ointment.

Where communal thermometers are used for recording skin temperature, care must be taken to ensure that they are immersed in a suitable disinfectant for an adequate length of time before using for the next patient. Savlon 1 in 30 in 70 per cent spirit for a minimum period of two minutes is recommended. The thermometer must be dried carefully.

To Record a Rectal Temperature

Requirements as above and, in addition, a container with petroleum jelly.

METHOD. The procedure is explained to the older child and assurance given that it is painless. He should be covered as this procedure can be embarrassing to sensitive children. The child is turned on his side; the infant can be held on the nurse's knee with his legs raised. The thermometer is wiped dry and shaken down to below 35°C or 95°F. The bulb is lubricated lightly and the thermometer is inserted into the rectum. The distance the thermometer is inserted is most important. If the bulb only is inserted, a skin temperature will be recorded which is up to 0·5C or 1-2°F less than rectal temperature. In an infant, the thermometer is inserted a full inch and, in the older child, 1½ inches. The thermometer must be held firmly by the nurse and the buttocks are lightly compressed for the period prescribed on the thermometer. The temperature is read and recorded. The thermometer is then washed and replaced in the disinfectant. The nurse washes and dries her hands. Rectal thermometers should be for individual use only.

Temperature Monitor

Temperature may be recorded by skin, oesophagus or rectum. To record a skin temperature, the thermister is attached with adhesive to any point of dry skin. Cottonwool placed between the thermister and the adhesive ensures effective insulation from outside temperatures.

To record the temperature in the oesophagus, the thermister is lubricated with a substance such as KY jelly and passed to a mid-point taken between the nape of the nose and the distal part of the xiphisternum. The thermister can be attached to the cheek with adhesive tape. To record the temperature in the rectum, the thermister is lubricated and passed 1-1½ inches.

RECORDING THE PULSE RATE

The child should be at rest either sitting on a chair or bed. It is pointless to attempt to count a pulse when a child has been running about in the ward or is distressed by crying.

The radial pulse is felt on the anterior aspect of the wrist; the arm should be supported and relaxed, the nurse feeling for the pulse with her first two fingers. It is recorded for one minute. The rate is counted and it is important to consider the character of the pulse and report any abnormality or irregularity of the beat.

Distraction for the toddler will be essential and usually he can be fascinated by the ticking of a watch. A pulse can be felt at the front of the ear or at the temple. In an infant the anterior fontanelle may have a visible pulse beat. It is helpful to record the pulse of an infant or toddler when he is asleep, it can otherwise be very difficult to obtain an accurate record of his pulse rate. Cot sides should therefore not be taken down and the child should be disturbed as little as possible until the pulse and respiration rates have been obtained; warm hands are necessary when feeling the pulse. The temperature in such instances would be recorded last.

To Record an Apical Heart Beat

This may be necessary when it is difficult to record the pulse rate accurately by digital means; also in some diseases the radial count is an inaccurate measurement of the actual heart beat.

The point of maximum cardiac impulse varies considerably. In a normal sized heart the apex beat can be heard in an infant in the third or fourth intercostal space, just outside the nipple line.

From 2-5 years: The fourth intercostal space at the nipple line.
Over 5 years: The fifth intercostal space, at or within the nipple line.

The apex beat may be visible. It is most accurately recorded by using a stethoscope. The child should be at rest. The diaphragm of the stethoscope is warmed by rubbing it with the hand. It is then placed over the point of maximum cardiac impulse and the rate recorded for one minute.

Pulse Rate Monitor

This is useful when recording pulse rates of over 140 beats per minute. The transducer can be attached to the forehead of a small infant.

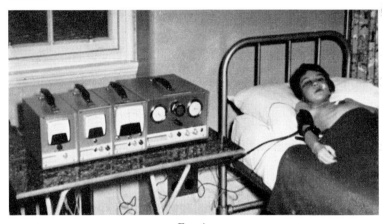

FIG. 1

Monitor recording temperature, pulse, respiration and blood pressure of a 7-year-old patient. An oesophageal thermister is being used. (The equipment is Air-Shields Inc.)

RECORDING THE RESPIRATORY RATE

This is not normally a difficult task, but it must be remembered that the older child may well effect an abnormal rate of respiration when being obviously watched. It is not sufficient to count the rate, observation must be made of the type and character of the respirations. This can only be adequately carried out by examining the bared chest. Respirations are counted for one minute. Any indrawing of the intercostal muscles above the manubrium sterni and excessive use of the abdominal muscles must be noted and reported.

Respiration Rate Monitor

This will record up to a rate of 90 per minute. The transducer is attached with adhesive tape to the patient's chest.

An APNOEA MONITOR is available (Air-Shields, U.K., Ltd.). This monitor can provide constant respiratory surveillance for the small infant; an early warning system operates when a pre-selected period of time elapses in which a baby has not taken a breath.

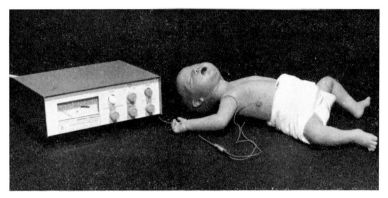

FIG. 1A
Apnoea monitor. (By kind permission of Air-Shields (U.K.) Ltd.)

TAKING AND RECORDING BLOOD PRESSURE

Blood pressure means the lateral pressure of the blood against the walls of the vessel which contains it. Clinically, the taking of blood pressure refers to the arterial pressure, usually in the brachial artery. In any individual, arterial pressure is not constant, but subject to variation over short intervals of time.

It is of diagnostic value and is indicative of progress or deterioration in certain conditions such as shock, head injury where there is increased intracranial pressure, kidney or heart disease. In the child, hypertension may occur in blood loss due to an over-compensating mechanism. When the fall in blood pressure occurs, it is sudden and dramatic. Excitement and struggling will increase the systolic pressure as much as 50 mm. Hg above the usual level. It is therefore important to have the child calm and quiet.

Blood pressure depends on:

(a) The strength of the contractions of the heart.

(b) The condition of the walls of the blood vessels.

(c) The amount of circulating blood.

(d) The viscosity of the blood.

Two pressures are measured:

1. Systolic, which is the higher one, due to the contractions of the heart muscle.

2. Diastolic, which is the lower one and is the pressure exerted on the arterial walls by the blood during rest.

The instrument used is known as a sphygmomanometer. It consists of an inflatable armlet which is fitted round the arm in the region of the brachial artery. The side tube of the armlet is connected to the mercury manometer.

REQUIREMENTS:

1. Sphygmomanometer with cuffs.

2. Stethoscope.

METHOD. The procedure should be explained to the older child and the smaller child is reassured. The child is lying flat and the arm band is wound round the arm above the elbow. The sphygmomanometer must be on a flat surface beside the child. The bag is inflated with air until it is just sufficient to obliterate the pulse. The point at which the pulse disappears is noted. On slight deflation of the bag, the pulse will return, and this is noted as the systolic pressure. A stethoscope is placed over the brachial artery and the bag is slowly deflated. The sound changes from a sharp tapping to a softer blowing noise and finally disappears. In most hospitals, the diastolic pressure is taken at the point when the sound changes to a softer blowing noise, but the more accurate point is when the sound disappears. The nurse therefore should ascertain from the medical staff which method is to be used.

Method of Taking the Blood Pressure of an Infant

In the infant the procedure is carried out by the doctor. It is more difficult to take and record the blood pressure of infants, therefore a more accurate method is the 'Flush' method. Here a small sphygmomanometer cuff is applied above the wrist or ankle. A crepe pressure bandage is wound round the hand or foot starting distally. The cuff is then inflated. When the bandage is removed, the limb will be white. The pressure in the cuff is reduced slowly and the point noted at which blood re-enters the limb causing flushing.

REQUIREMENTS:

1. Sphygmomanometer with a small cuff.
2. Crepe bandage.
3. Stethoscope.

Blood Pressure Monitor

Systolic and diastolic blood pressures are recorded on separate dials. Readings may be taken automatically on a 2-minute or a 4-minute cycle or at any other time.

Such equipment is of immense value for obtaining accurate recordings, particularly in the case of very ill children when they may be otherwise very difficult to obtain.

RECORDING OF VITAL SIGNS OF CHILDREN WITH HEAD INJURY

Children recover more rapidly from head injury and are less likely to suffer permanent cerebral damage than adults. The post-accident period, however, is fraught with as many dangers, and careful observation and assessment of condition is essential.

The frequency with which vital signs are recorded is dependent on the condition of the child. It may be necessary for the child to have constant nursing care with half-hourly or hourly recording of signs.

A definition of level of consciousness is necessary. It is then appropriate to record only a single word on the chart. The definitions given have been adapted from those used in the Department of Surgical Neurology, Royal Infirmary, Edinburgh.

Description of Level of Consciousness

1. *Mild.* The child, though confused in some degree, is capable of coherent conversation and appropriate behaviour. He sits up in bed but may be inattentive and irritable and cry readily.

2. *Moderate.* The child, though out of touch with his surroundings, may give relevant answers to simple questions, such as 'What is your name?' 'How old are you?' 'Where do you live?' He prefers to be left alone, sleeps most of the time and may resent disturbance and be very irritable.

3. *Severe.* Child mostly inaccessible, but sometimes responds to simple, forceful commands; e.g. 'Put out your tongue', 'Grip my hand'. Resists attention, and may fight or speak incoherently, giving angry cries if hurt. Can assume a comfortable position. Pupils often equal and reactive. Change in size, especially with impairment of light reflex, is important.

4. *Semicoma.* Postural tone present. Respiration shallow or stertorous. Responds to painful stimuli by movement but no response to verbal stimuli. Pupils may be unequal, open or contracted, may respond to light. Corneal reflex present. Swallowing may be present but no attempt made to feed. Urinary incontinence with reflex emptying.

5. *Coma.* Postural tone lost but decerebrate rigidity may be present. No response even to painful stimuli. Pupils dilated, do not react to light. Corneal reflexes absent. Cannot swallow or cough. Will drown in his own secretions, if left flat on his back.

OTHER SIGNS

It will be necessary also to record the state of the pupils and ears. Abbreviations could be as follows:

Pupils	*Ears*
C—contracted	N—Normal
M—medium	B—Blood discharge
D—dilated	S—Serous discharge
F—fixed	
N—normal	

A chart can be designed for recording all these signs, and in addition pulse, blood pressure, and respiration rates.

RECORDING VITAL SIGNS OF CHILDREN WITH CONVULSIONS

The young child has a low threshold for convulsions and it is, therefore, not an uncommon manifestation of illness. It may arise when the child is hyperpyrexic and dehydrated, such as after excessive exposure to the sun, or it may herald the onset of a severe infective illness or cerebral episode. It is, therefore, important for the nurse to note exactly:

1. The duration of the convulsion.
2. The nature of the movement: clonic—spasm with successive muscular contractions and relaxations; tonic—with continuous muscular contractions.
3. The extent of the movement, also which limbs involved, which part of the body, face or eyes.
4. The conscious level and any other relevant information such as incontinence, child's condition before and after the convulsion.

An observation chart is necessary. The type which provides for anecdotal comment is to be preferred. The temperature, pulse and respiration should be recorded and charted following the episode.

FLUID AND ELECTROLYTE BALANCE

The child's response to imbalance can be sudden and severe. His body reserves do not permit delay. Early recognition of signs and accurate record keeping are essential. The smaller the child the greater the urgency.

The extent of electrolyte imbalance can be assessed from the venous blood and corrected by the judicious use of the appropriate fluid. An infant has a circulating blood volume of 400 to 500 ml. compared with an adult, who has 5 to 6 litres. It will be appreciated that great accuracy is required in giving the correct amount of fluid in the stated time.

A standard 24-hour chart used throughout the hospital lessens the risk of error and confusion when nurses in training move from ward to ward. Only abbreviations printed on the chart should be used. Numerals should be in columns, one digit one column for ease of counting (Fig. 2). A simple digital adding machine is a valuable asset.

Assessment of the amount of urine or vomit which cannot be measured is difficult. If stated as small, medium, or large, the assessment of the amount can be made by the person responsible for maintaining the balance.

Assessment of fluid lost in bowel movements is of vital importance with infants who have diarrhoea. A baby can collapse very suddenly through loss of fluid without having had any vomiting.

24 HOUR INTAKE OUTPUT CHART

Name: Jean Smith   Starting at: 9 a.m. p.m. on ____   Ward 2 ____

Weight: 8·18 Kg.

Time	INTAKE		OUTPUT			Drugs*
	Food and Fluids	Amount Given - ml	Urine ml	Vomit or Aspirate-ml	Stool	Nature and Amount
9 a.m.	MILK	1 2 0	6 0			
10 a.m.						
11 a.m.						
12 noon Dinner						
1 p.m.						

FIG. 2

Fluid balance chart—note the one digit, one column for greater accuracy and easier addition.

Potassium deficiency can occur when a child is vomiting, or when gastric aspirations are continued over several days. Potassium will be lost from the stomach as well as from the urine. The child will be seen to be cross, irritable, and apathetic; there will be loss of muscle tone.

It is important to understand this is a manifestation of the illness which can be corrected once the electrolyte balance is achieved. Signs of over-hydration require to be carefully watched for. Dependent oedema will be apparent and, providing the kidneys are functioning adequately, the urinary output will be observed to increase.

BIBLIOGRAPHY

Bendall, E. R. D. & Raybould, E. (1965). *Basic Nursing*, 2nd ed. London: Lewis.

Blake, G. F. & Wright, H. F. (1963). *Essentials of Paediatrics*. London: Pitman.

British Medical Association (1966). *Child Care*. Commissioned Articles. London: B.M.A.

Ellis, R. W. B. (1966). *Child Health and Development*, 4th ed. London: Churchill.

Gainsborough, H. (1962). *Nurs. Times*, **58**, 697, 737.

CHAPTER III

WARD INFECTION

Sources of infection and mode of spread; dangers of the spread of infection; aspects in the prevention of the spread of infection.

INFECTION is the successful invasion, establishment and growth of micro organisms in the tissues of the host (from Livingstone's Dictionary for Nurses).

SOURCES OF INFECTION AND MODE OF SPREAD

The source of an infection occurring in a ward originates from the people therein: either patient, visitor, or member of the staff. Such a person may be:

(*a*) Known to have an infection.

(*b*) In the incubation period of a disease and, therefore, symptom-free, but in an infectious state.

(*c*) A carrier. A person who is convalescent from an infectious illness, or one who is symptom-free but harbours the organism and can transmit infection to others.

(*d*) A patient who has been misdiagnosed. This may arise when there is a confusion of symptoms, or when these are so mild as to give no cause for concern.

The mode of spread of infection from such sources can be:

(*a*) RESPIRATORY: The organisms are inspired. In many diseases the organisms responsible are present in the saliva or nasal secretions; e.g. Pneumococcus, and in sputum; e.g. Tubercle bacillus.

(*b*) GASTRO-INTESTINAL—FAECES: The organisms are swallowed with contaminated food, water or dust. There are many different strains causing gastro-enteritis. The *Escherichia coli* is particularly virulent to infants, but rarely causes symptoms in the older child though he may become a short-term carrier.

(c) CUTANEOUS: Where there is a break in the skin, organisms can enter from septic skin lesions, wounds, burns or abscesses; the *Staphylococcus aureus* is normally found on the skin of ward staff. It is a common causative organism of infected lesions. Transmission from such sources can be by:

(a) CONTACT either direct or indirect. Hands if not washed adequately are considered to be the main cause of transmission of infection from the gastro-intestinal tract and skin surfaces. The nails and nailbeds harbour germs. Clothes coming in contact with an infectious person; also linen, blankets, toys and all communal equipment may transmit organisms. Food and milk, or crockery and cutlery, may easily become a vehicle for transmission of infection. Houseflies are dangerous carriers and their access to food or milk must be prevented at all times by adequate covering and proper storage.

(b) DROPLET INFECTION: Organisms from the nasopharynx are sent into the air during normal respiration. During coughing, talking or sneezing they may be projected as much as six feet. Transmission of pathogenic organisms can occur this way directly into an open wound, or on to some article which may transmit the organism later, such as pathogenic organisms breathed on to instruments or dressings. Pathogenic organisms breathed into the atmosphere will also contribute to the infectivity of dust and the bacterial content of the atmosphere.

DANGERS OF THE SPREAD OF INFECTION

The dangers must be realised by all those whose responsibility it is to care for the infant and young child in hospital. An ill child will have lowered resistance to infection and the infant whose immunity is not yet fully developed is at very considerable risk. It is not enough for a routine to be laid down. With pressure of work and lack of understanding, this may not be maintained. One careless or thoughtless action can ruin the work of a whole team. A chain is only as strong as its weakest link. It is, therefore, essential that all members of the team should understand how infection can be spread and the consequences of any such spread.

Many micro organisms can cause infection and there is a variety of ways in which infection can spread. The Staphylococcus is one of the organisms which has become an increasing danger in hospitals over the past few years. It is used here as an example to demonstrate the consequences of spread of infection and to emphasise to those caring for the sick child the importance of knowing how infection spreads and the precautions which must be taken to prevent such spread.

It has been found that babies born in hospital become carriers of coagulase positive Staphylococci (i.e. *Staphylococcus aureus*) very soon after birth, and may retain these Staphylococci for many months. When we consider that these organisms may produce serious results, the grave concern felt should make us critically review our techniques and procedures in the light of present-day knowledge and research.

When a clean wound becomes infected, some technique has been faulty and somehow infection has been introduced. This may appear obvious but no less real is the spread of infection which occurs when the baby in the neonatal period develops a septic focus leading to a more serious condition; e.g. osteomyelitis, pneumonia and septicaemia. Cross infection may also occur when one infant or child develops a lesion from another. Such infection can spread from a 'sticky' eye, an infected umbilicus, or a tiny septic nailbed.

The original source is not so easy to locate but no member of staff or visitor should be handling infants if they have any infected lesion however small.

Staphylococcal pneumonia may result after the organism has been lying dormant in the nares for months. Babies with pneumonia can be desperately ill and exceptionally difficult to treat. As with neonatal osteomyelitis, the organisms are usually bred in hospital and, therefore, resistant to many if not all of the antibiotics in common use. Unless scientists can keep ahead and produce new antibiotics as organisms become resistant to the old ones, we will be in a situation such as existed before penicillin was discovered when there was no weapon to fight the infection. With a few unfortunate children, this is indeed the case. The children have chronic foci, which do not respond to existing drugs.

The Staphylococcus is not the only organism which can be spread, nor are the examples quoted the only results of infection, but such examples do demonstrate the consequences and make us realise the importance of knowing what precautions we must take to prevent cross infection.

ASPECTS IN THE PREVENTION OF THE
SPREAD OF INFECTION

Education

The most important factor in the prevention of the spread of infection is the understanding by all members of the staff of the dangers involved, the sources of spread, and of measures which can be adopted to prevent such infection.

Constant review of methods and techniques is necessary. All members of the nursing staff should read the current literature: The Control of Cross Infection in Hospital, M.R.C. memorandum; Staphylococcal Infection in Hospital, report of the Subcommittee Central Health Services Council Standing Medical Advisory Committee, H.M.S.O.

Discussion with all the ward staff is essential. A routine should be evolved for the care of infants and small children which can be carried out by the existing staff. The orderly and ward maid require to be included when teaching cleanliness and hygiene. They must have a proper understanding of the requirements; otherwise, it will be found that dishes will be sterilised only on occasion, or 'after dinner to remove the grease better'. They must understand the danger of dust and the importance of using the correct equipment and not fall back on the sweeping brush because they do not understand new-fangled machines and have not had them properly demonstrated; suction cleaners reduce the amount of dust rising into the atmosphere, providing the filter is changed at regular intervals, and are, therefore, greatly to be preferred.

Disinfection is an essential part of preventive measures. It is not given priority in sequence because it is more important than other aspects, but merely because it has a bearing on them.

Prevention of contamination must always be the aim.

The use of disposable items, which can be used once and disposed of safely and promptly in closed containers, is an important contributary factor in our preventative measures, but staff require instruction in their use and disposal. To leave such items lying in the ward, or in open containers after use, is surely to defeat their value.

WASTE DISPOSABLE UNITS with paper sacks (Permapure) are of value. When the sack is removed it is automatically sealed.

Syringes and Needles require particular care in their disposal. Needles may perforate paper sacks and cause injury to the collector of waste. Syringes found by children may be used as playthings, or may be used by drug addicts. Serum Hepatitis is one grave danger of such misuse. It is therefore essential to ensure that such syringes and needles are not available to the public. It is advocated by some that the syringe is broken and the needle bent immediately after use. This is unnecessary if arrangements can be made with the local council that they be collected from a locked container in the hospital grounds and incinerated without any direct handling.

Disinfection

Disinfection is the means by which bacteria are rendered harmless. Various methods of disinfection can be used; these include heat (dry and moist heat), spray disinfection of air, ultra-violet radiation, gamma rays, and chemical disinfection.

Chemical disinfectants are a useful tool, and there is a wide choice available. It is essential that, whatever the choice, they must be used with care. It must be understood that all chemical disinfectants are to some extent active against bacteria, but will not destroy organisms such as tubercle bacilli and fungi. A chemical disinfectant should not be used where more effective methods are available; e.g. crockery, linen and bedpans are more effectively sterilised by heat. When chemical disinfection is the choice, consideration must be given to the following points:

(*a*) Behaviour of disinfectants; e.g. some disinfectants are inactivated by soap, or when diluted with hard water.

(*b*) Efficiency in killing bacteria. Different dilutions of one particular disinfectant may be recommended for different purposes.

(*c*) It should be non-caustic, non-corrosive to fabric and where possible be kind to the hands. Care should be taken to avoid skin reactions.

(*d*) A disinfectant will be more effective if as much organic matter as possible is removed before the disinfectant is applied; e.g. a bedpan should be washed before applying a disinfectant.

(*e*) A reasonable time must be allowed for any disinfectant to

C

do its work. It is useless to expect disinfection to occur by dipping an item into the disinfectant for a few seconds. The manufacturers give guidance on this point with their products.

(f) Disinfectants should always be freshly made up to the required strength in containers which have been sterilised by heat. This is due to the fact that micro-organisms are able to survive and multiply in quite strong solutions when left standing for any length of time.

Suggested types and strengths can be found in the appendix.

Design

Well designed equipment with smooth surfaces which can be readily cleaned and sterilised or disinfected is necessary.

Consideration should also be given to furnishings which should be simple and readily laundered. Ward toys, like ward equipment and furniture, should be well designed with smooth surfaces. Advice and help in ward design furniture, furnishings, and equipment can be obtained from the Hospital Centres in London and Edinburgh.

Visitors

It has not been proved that visitors bring more infection into the ward than do members of the staff, and parents are a very necessary part of a child's life in hospital. They must, however, understand that if there is any infection or illness in the home, advice should be sought from the sister as to the advisability of visiting. The benefit of children maintaining contact with their brothers and sisters must be weighed against the dangers of possible transmission of one of the childhood ailments, such as measles, mumps or chicken-pox. Known infection at school or in the district should be notified to sister. Minor coughs and colds which may not upset an adult can be serious if passed on to an ill child about to have an anaesthetic, and again in such circumstances the desirability of visiting must be discussed with sister.

Staff

Staff must also appreciate the harm which they may do if they persist in staying on duty infecting others with their ailments.

The Staphylococcus may be transmitted from one person to another from a septic focus, however minor. A sore throat may be the sign of streptococcal infection and such an infection can be very harmful if transmitted to others, especially infants already weakened with another illness. Diarrhoea is a significant symptom which should never go unregarded when working with children.

It is, therefore, not noble to be a martyr and stay on duty, but much wiser to report such symptoms and have them treated before the infection spreads.

Ventilation

Ventilation means the exchange of impure air for pure air without causing draughts. The importance of good ventilation in hospital cannot be over-emphasised in an endeavour to keep the bacterial content of the air at a minimum and thus reduce the risk of spread of infection. Ventilation can be obtained by the simple method of opening windows and ensuring that there are no unpleasant draughts. This may not be satisfactory if the air outside is impure, or if it is not at the desired temperature. Air-conditioning plants can maintain a desired temperature and humidity; an air change six times per hour is recommended (Hospital Building Notes).

Elimination of Overcrowding

Understanding and co-operation at all levels can do much to relieve this situation. Overcrowding means not only that patients are too near each other, but that there is lack of equipment for them, and lack of staff to look after them. All the factors add up to the danger of spread of infection. When there is lack of staff and people are overworked, there is not time to give adequate nursing care. The recommendation from the Hospital Building Notes is that beds and cots should be at 8 ft. centres with sufficient space between the foot ends to ensure passage of other beds or portable equipment.

Communal Surfaces

Obviously when trying to prevent the spread of infection, communal surfaces are open to grave criticism and should be avoided whenever possible. Such things as baby baths should be cleaned thoroughly between bathings. The disinfectant must be used correctly remembering that the length of exposure to the disinfectant is as important as the strength. The dangerous practice of drying a surface immediately it has been washed and before the disinfectant has had time to act is to be deprecated. Disposable cloths are to be recommended.

Disposable sheets are available and can be used on examination couches and weighing scales. They are used once only and are then discarded.

All equipment which cannot be adequately disinfected must be avoided.

Communal toys for babies and toddlers are a danger. An infant frequently puts things into his mouth and, therefore, babies' toys must be clean and not handed from one to another without adequate disinfection.

Hand-washing

Infection can be spread from unwashed hands and everyone has a part to play in ensuring that this is understood. Notices in lavatories and other places are not enough.

Nail brushes have a questionable value and if used with excessive zeal open hacks and nail-beds, providing a site for infection giving rise to paronychiae. Repeated use of a nail brush stored in disinfectant is dangerous. Organisms such as the *Pseudomonas pyocyanea* have been found to flourish in such receptacles. Nail brushes, if required, should be packed in a dispenser and sterilised by autoclaving at 134°C for 3 minutes.

Hands should be washed under a running tap for a full minute and dried carefully on a disposable towel or by hot air. A communal ward towel is a source of infection (Fig. 3).

Chemical disinfectants are available which endeavour to render the hands free from organisms. There is a risk of skin reaction with all chemical disinfectants and skin sensitivity must be considered when trying any new preparation. Antibacterial washing creams containing $2\frac{1}{2}$ per cent hexachlorophane; dispensers with hexachlorophane soap leaves, and a providone iodine preparation containing $\frac{3}{4}$ per cent available iodine have all proved efficacious. Gillespie *et al.* (1962) and Williams *et al.* (1966) state that the *Staphylococcus aureus* on nurses' hands was less numerous when hexachlorophane soap was regularly used, or chlorhexidine cream applied after drying. This has been confirmed by the authors.

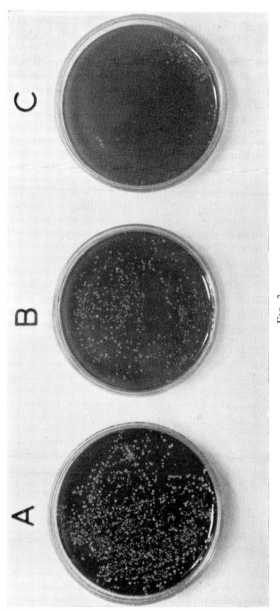

FIG. 3

Hand-washing. Agar plates 24 hours after inoculation with swabs taken from (A) hands before washing, (B) hands after washing and drying with communal ward towel, (C) hands after washing and drying with a paper hand towel.

It is essential that taps should be operated by elbow or foot pedal and not touched by infected hands.

Hand-washing does not render the hands sterile. Therefore, procedures requiring an aseptic technique demand the use of sterile forceps. Contaminated linen, or other infected substances should not be handled. Handling should be reduced to the minimum, but if this is necessary gloves can be worn and disposable gloves are available for this purpose.

Specific times of hand-washing cannot all be laid down here, but the following times should be considered as essential (after Williams *et al.*, 1966).

1. On arrival and before leaving the ward.
2. Before and after any procedure for which gloves or forceps are necessary, or any procedure requiring sterilised equipment.
3. After any item of service for a patient, who is, or should be, isolated.
4. Before and after washing a baby, cleaning its eyes, nose or mouth, changing a napkin, or dressing the umbilicus.
5. After rounds of temperature-taking, bed-making, and bed-pans.
6. Before preparing food or infants' feeds.
7. After defaecation and at other times when contamination seems especially likely.

Gowns

To be of any value, these must be properly put on and worn correctly. It must be understood why they should be worn, and that they are not merely garments for keeping a uniform clean. It is important to prevent the nurse's uniform coming in contact with the patient or his linen thereby transmitting infection from one child to the other through the medium of the uniform.

It is necessary, therefore, to wear a gown when giving any nursing care to a patient who has an infection which may be transmitted to others. It is also considered important to wear a gown when giving nursing care to infants to prevent transmission of infection to them from the nurse's uniform. In all instances, it is essential that a separate gown is worn for each child. This should be hung on a hanger at the child's bed and renewed every twenty-four hours or more often if necessary (Fig. 4).

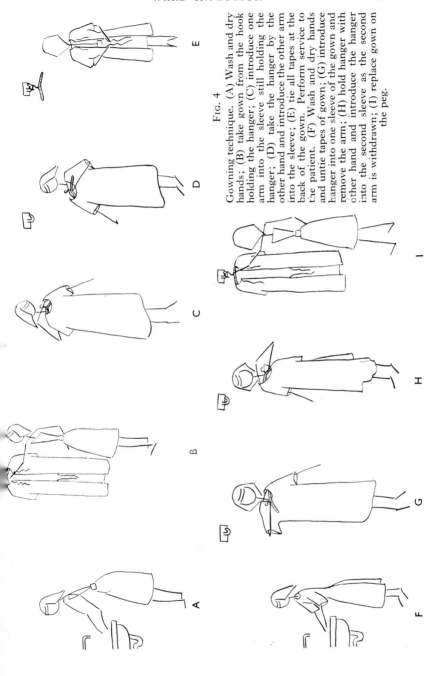

FIG. 4

Gowning technique. (A) Wash and dry hands; (B) take gown from the hook holding the hanger; (C) introduce one arm into the sleeve still holding the hanger; (D) take the hanger by the other hand and introduce the other arm into the sleeve; (E) tie all tapes at the back of the gown. Perform service to tie patient. (F) Wash and dry hands and untie tapes of gown; (G) introduce hanger into one sleeve of the gown and remove the arm; (H) hold hanger with other hand and introduce the hanger into the second sleeve as the second arm is withdrawn; (I) replace gown on the peg.

Masks

There are many opinions held as to the advisability of wearing masks, but agreement is readily reached on the dangers of not wearing a mask properly. A mask reduces the number of organisms projected into the atmosphere during speech, and it is, therefore, advocated by many that they should be used in the following circumstances:

1. When preparing for, and carrying out a procedure which requires an aseptic technique.
2. When attending premature or weak infants.
3. When the nurse, or patient being cared for, has a respiratory infection.

It is obvious that the mask must harbour organisms shortly after it is worn and to prevent it being a source of spread of infection certain rules must be observed.

Rules for wearing masks :

1. Masks should not be touched while being worn.
2. The mask should be changed when it becomes moist.
3. The mask should not be loose. It must be well fitting.
4. The mask when removed must be touched only by the tapes or elastic and placed immediately into a container with a lid.

Handling of the gauze or paper part of the mask when it is on will contaminate the hands and render them a source of infection.

The length of time a mask may be worn and be considered a safe barrier is difficult to determine. No mask can provide even for a short time a safe barrier if the wearer has a heavy cold. Providing that the wearer does not have a heavy cold or is not perspiring freely, the two-ply type disposable mask can be worn in all probability effectively for one to two hours (Smith and Nephew, Southalls Ltd. recommendation). The gauze mask is apparently effective for a period of up to three hours (research for Robinson and Sons Ltd., Chesterfield by C. G. A. Thomas, Department of Clinical Pathology, Guy's Hospital).

Disposable paper masks are ideal for use in the ward, but the supply of these must be adequate, and suitable containers for used masks should be conveniently placed.

Care of the Young Infant

The infant in the first few weeks of life is at a most vulnerable period when immunity is not fully developed. Precautions, therefore, must be taken to prevent all possible risk of infection. These babies whenever possible should be isolated in cubicles; the alternative is to ensure they have all their own equipment beside them in the open ward. They should be positioned beside a hand basin and a strict hand-washing regime observed.

Making of Feeds

This is a specialised task, which should be carried out under as aseptic conditions as possible. Ideally, the milk kitchen should be apart from the ward, with its own staff who have no contact with the ward.

In many hospitals, terminal sterilisation has been instituted. With this method, feeds are made up in the usual way, the teats are then put on the bottles, and over these are put shields, or paper cones. The bottles are then numbered and dated, and finally sterilised. With this method, the infant does not have the same teat each time and it may be necessary to supply additional teats in separate sterile packs.

Bulk food mixers as made by Cow and Gate and Glaxo Laboratories are most useful for small paediatric units or maternity units where there is not a wide range of feeds. They eliminate a considerable amount of routine work and, therefore, can effect economy in staff. A milk dispenser for use with canned milk has been designed, incorporating the use of disposable feeding bottles (Michelson, A.). This unit would be most satisfactory where there is not a wide range of feeds.

Infant Feeding Routine

To ensure the least risk of transmitting infection to the infant, it is necessary to plan a routine suitable for the circumstances and equipment available in the hospital. The more simple the routine, the more likely will it be carried out. It is difficult to reduce the number of times hands have to be washed but careful drying and the use of hand creams will be helpful in the prevention of sore hands. The use of a barrier cream is an additional precaution advocated by many.

Example. The following routine is both simple and straight-forward:

1. The nurse washes and dries her hands, puts on a gown, and changes the infant. The soiled napkin is left in a closed container. Hands are washed and dried and the gown removed.

2. The name on the feeding bottle is checked to ensure that each infant is given the correct feed. It is heated and taken to the bedside, the teat being kept carefully covered. The hands are washed and dried, the gown is put on and the infant fed. The infant is changed again if necessary and the hands are washed and dried before removing the gown.

3. The feeding bottle is taken to the kitchen. It is carried in one hand, the other being left free to open doors. The receptacle for heating the feed is put into a container for disinfection. The bottle and teat are then washed carefully to remove all particles of milk and are then submerged in a 1:80 solution of sodium hypochlorite (Milton) for $1\frac{1}{2}$ hours. It is important not to lay anything down on a communal surface which may cause spread of infection from the infant.

The use of disposable bottles and teats eliminates any problems associated with immersing large numbers of bottles and teats for the required period of time.

Electric warmers are useful and eliminate such hazards as over-heated feeds or containers with boiling water which could be spilled. However, they create an obvious problem of adequate disinfection and when used it is recommended that they be kept in the infant's cubicle and not carried from one bedside to another.

The soiled napkin and the linen are then disposed of, and the final washing and drying of the hands takes place.

Toilet Round

When it is remembered that faeces may contain disease-producing organisms, then it should be understood that bedpans must be considered as a source of infection and, therefore, always sterilised after use. A bedpan steriliser with steam jets or boiling for three minutes is adequate for routine disinfection.

If bedpans are taken round by trolley, two trolleys are required. It is essential that clean bedpans are not contaminated by being laid on a surface which has had a used bedpan. A difficulty can arise with the use of disposable bedpans. When the disposing cycle is in progress, contaminated bedpans cannot immediately be disposed of and any area they are laid upon must be considered contaminated.

Bedpan covers must not be transferred from one bedpan to another; disposable covers are available. Toilet gowns should be changed frequently; it is desirable to have one gown for each toilet round. If contaminated, or wet, it should be changed immediately.

Hand-washing routine must be carried out after dealing with a bedpan. Children who go to the toilet or deal with their own cleansing when on bedpans must be given the opportunity to wash their hands afterwards.

Regular servicing with scrupulous cleanliness and disinfection of children's toilets is necessary.

Observation and Reporting

The importance of observing and reporting immediately any sign and symptom cannot be overstressed. The young baby who normally feeds well and suddenly loses interest in his feeds, or the toddler who rejects his dinner and just wants to curl up and go to sleep, may well be displaying the first signs of infection and these should be noted before there is any dramatic change from a normal temperature or local evidence of spread of infection. There must be no hesitation in reporting such signs. Infection is less likely to spread when everyone is on the watch and adequate precautions are taken early.

These points are guiding principles only. In the prevention of spread of infection individual hospitals will plan their methods to suit circumstances, but the principles are the same, and if understood, providing equipment is adequate, they can and must be observed.

BIBLIOGRAPHY

Dennison, W. M. (1968). *Surgery in Infancy and Childhood*, 2nd ed. Edinburgh: Livingstone.
Harmer, B. & Henderson, V. (1955). *Principles and Practice of Nursing*, 5th ed. New York: Macmillan.
Mauras, I. M. (1968). *Nurs. Mirror*, **126**, 25.
Medical Research Council (1951). *The Control of Cross Infection in Hospital*. London: H.M.S.O.

Michelson, A. (1966). Disposable feeding bottles. *Nurs. Times*, **62**, 44.

Ministry of Health (1959). *Central Health Council Report on Staphylococcal Infection in Hospital.* London: H.M.S.O.

Ministry of Health (1964). *Children's Ward.* Hospital Building Notes 23. London: H.M.S.O.

Nuffield Provincial Trust (1959). *Sterilising Practice in Six Hospitals.*

Nursing Times (1966). Cross infection control in hospitals. Hospital Centre Report. *Nurs. Times*, **62**, 51.

Nursing Times (1966). The proper use of a mask. *Nurs. Times*, **62**, 45.

Rubbo, S. D. & Gardner, J. F. (1965). *A Review of Sterilisation and Disinfection.* London: Lloyd Luke.

Williams, R. E. O., Blowers, R., Garrod, L. P. & Shotter, R. A. (1966). *Hospital Infection*, 2nd ed. London: Lloyd Luke.

CHAPTER IV

NURSING CARE OF THE PREMATURE INFANT

Characteristics of premature infants; preservation of body temperature; preparation of incubator and cot; care of the incubator; prevention of infection; handling of the infant; feeding of the infant; preparation for dismissal.

THE nursing of premature babies is a responsible and exacting task. Meticulous attention to detail of observation and technique is absolutely essential to give the infant every possible chance of development. By international standards a baby weighing 5½ lb. (2,500 grammes) or less at birth is termed premature regardless of the period of gestation.

Characteristics of Premature Infants

The characteristics vary with the foetal age. The larger premature infant of 4-5½ lb. (1·8 kg.-2·5 kg.) is usually active, whereas the smaller infant whose weight is below 4 lb. (1·8 kg.) shows little activity and has a feeble, infrequent cry. The respirations tend to be irregular in rhythm and depth and periods of apnoea with cyanosis may occur. The cough reflex is absent in the smaller infants, increasing the danger of inhalation of regurgitated fluids. The capacity of the stomach is small, the digestive powers are weak and the sucking and swallowing reflexes poorly developed. The skin is thin, red and wrinkled and there is very little subcutaneous fat. It is this factor as well as the relatively large surface area, muscular inactivity, inadequate sweating mechanism and an immature heat regulating centre which are largely responsible for the instability of body temperature.

Preservation of Body Temperature

The chances of survival of the premature infant are lessened if the body temperature is allowed to fall. Temperatures of premature infants in the first week of life may be as low as 33·3°C or 92°F. Rapid raising of body temperature is thought by some

paediatricians to be detrimental to the infant, because it increases
the basal metabolic rate and therefore, the oxygen requirements.
Once normal body temperature has been achieved (approx.
36·1-37·2°C or 97-99°F), which may not be until the second week

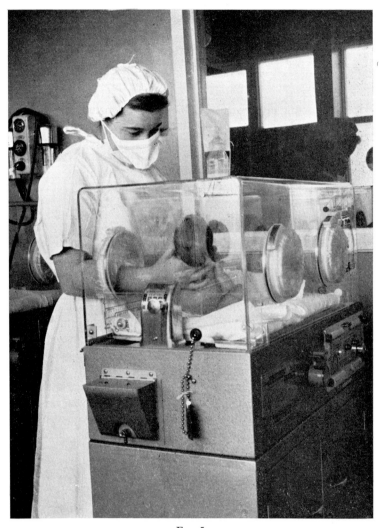

FIG. 5
Isolette. Incubator designed by Air-Shields Inc., showing the nurse supporting the infant.

of life, it is important to maintain it. Many different types of incubators can be used but none of them do away with the necessity of careful nursing and supervision. Bulbs and electric elements burn out and automatic thermostats sometimes fail, therefore, unless the incubator temperature and the temperature of the infant are checked frequently, harmful chilling or overheating may occur. A relative humidity of 70-80 per cent prevents dehydration and the ultimate irritant action of oxygen. The infant's temperature, taken 30 minutes after placement into the incubator, will determine subsequent regulation of the incubator temperature.

If the infant is to be nursed in an open cot, the temperature of the room should be maintained at 21·6-26·7°C or 70-80°F. The cot temperature should be maintained at 29·4-32·2°C or 85-90°F. Infants in an open cot can be dressed in light, warm clothing which will not interfere with their respiratory movements. The danger of overheating is very real and the cot should contain a thermometer, so that any variations can be observed and, therefore, rectified.

Preparation of the Incubator

Two types of incubators are in common use:

1. The 'opening' one which allows access to the child by opening the incubator lid.
2. The 'closed type' where the infant is nursed through 'sleeves' or windows (Fig. 5). These provide isolation for the infant from airborne infection but if used carelessly the sleeves can be a source of infection.

Before receiving the infant, the incubator is prewarmed to approximately 29·4°C or 85°F for infants of 1·7 kg. or 3½ lb. and 32·2°C or 90°F for the smaller infant. The tank is filled with three pints or approximately 2 litres of distilled or sterile distilled water and a napkin is placed on the foam mattress. The tray should contain the following:

1. Mucus extractor in container.
2. Destructible boxes with swabs, cotton wool balls, petroleum jelly.
3. Jar to hold a low-registering thermometer.
4. Receptacle for used swabs.

Oxygen supply should be available with the necessary rubber tubing and a flowmeter.

Preparation of the Cot

Various types of cots are used in hospitals. One of them is the Sorrento cot. This can be fitted with washable linings having three divisions which are large enough to hold hot water bottles. If oxygen is required a Perspex cover is placed over the cot and oxygen is given through a funnel from the oxygen supply. The end of the cot is provided with a small locker which contains the same articles as the incubator tray. Another type of cot is the Belfast cot which consists of a Perspex basket sitting on a trolley (Fig. 6). The advantage of this type is that the infant can be readily seen.

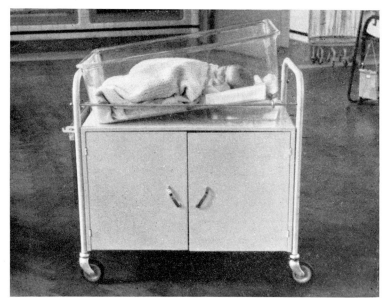

FIG. 6
Belfast cot

Administration of Oxygen

Oxygen is an important therapeutic aid. When it is administered to a premature baby, the nurse must bear in mind the dangers of retrolental fibroplasia with subsequent blindness. This can occur when the concentration of oxygen exceeds 40 per cent given over a long period. A slightly increased environmental oxygen has been shown to decrease the frequency and duration of apnoeic attacks in the premature baby. Higher levels of oxygen may be ordered where central cyanosis is present but it should not exceed 40 per cent over a long period. The oxygen concentration in an incubator or cot should be checked periodically by means of a reliable oxygen analyser. An analyser which is used and gives a reasonable degree of accuracy is the Mira Analyser (Fig. 7).

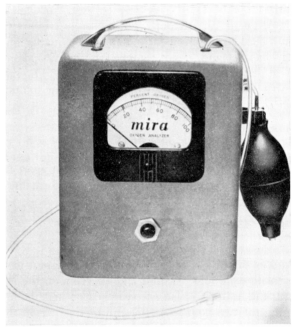

FIG. 7
Mira oxygen analyser. (By kind permission of Vickers Ltd.)

METHOD

The instrument is placed on a flat surface. The sample of oxygen is taken via a small section of polythene tubing which is suspended into the centre position of the treatment chamber through an aperture on the top. The aspirator bulb is deflated

4-6 times to obtain a sample of the oxygen mixture. When the bulb is fully inflated, the switch is pressed and held for 2-3 seconds.

Care of the Incubator

The outside of the incubator is cleaned daily. The tank is filled daily with fresh distilled or sterile water. Care is taken that the temperature of the water is approximately the same as that of the removed water and that adequate water is present at all times. Where sleeves are used they must provide an adequate seal.

When the infant is able to leave the incubator, thorough cleaning and disinfection is carried out. The mattress and tray are removed and cleaned. Vomitus, urine and faecal matter may enter the inner chamber and, if not removed as soon as possible, will harden and dry and can be a source of infection. The interior of the chamber should be washed with a disinfectant solution, such as a 2 per cent solution of Sudol.

The incubator can be fumigated as follows:

It is best carried out in a well ventilated room apart from the hospital wards, using a 5 per cent solution of formalin (40 per cent formaldehyde).

METHOD

The tank is drained and is then refilled with 1 pint or 600 ml. of the formalin solution. The lid and all vents on the incubator are closed; the heater and fan are switched on and the incubator left running for two hours. At the end of this period the water container should be emptied, washed out and 1 pint or 600 ml. of weak ammonia solution (approx. 0·05 per cent of 0·88 ammonia) put in. The incubator should then be run for a further period of 15 minutes with the lid and vents closed and the heater and fan switched on to enable the ammonia to neutralise residual formaldehyde. Finally, the ammonia solution should be emptied out. The interior of the nursing chamber is dried with a clean cloth, and the incubator left running for a short time with the lid and all vents open to get rid of any remaining smell.

ASPECTS OF PREVENTION OF INFECTION

1. Isolation

The premature infant has little or no resistance to infection and everyone who comes in contact with premature infants must be constantly aware of the danger of infection. Ideally these babies are isolated and have a special team of nurses to care for them. As few people as possible should enter the nursery and all should wear special gowns or dresses. Masks are worn for special procedures; e.g. exchange transfusion. No one with a cold, sore throat, skin lesions or other forms of infection should work in a premature baby unit. The furniture in the nursery is cleaned daily with a damp cloth and suction cleaners are used instead of sweeping. Blankets should be of the cotton variety which are economical in laundering, do not cause dust and can be boiled. All soiled linen pails must have lids and contain disposable bags or linings. After the pails are emptied, they are washed and disinfected. Neither clean nor dirty linen must come in contact with the nurse's uniform.

2. Hand-washing

Hand-washing cannot be stressed too greatly as a means of preventing spread of infection. Hands are washed before and after attending a baby, before the preparation of feeds and before putting on teats. Special provision should be made for drying the hands and disposable towels should be used. Hands must be dried thoroughly to prevent hacks and cracks of the skin which could provide an ideal surface for bacterial entry. A substance called hexachlorophane washing cream is most effective in inhibiting the growth of Staphylococci and is kind to the skin.

3. Masks

When a mask is worn, both the nose and mouth must be covered and it must not be handled while being worn. When removing the mask it is held by the tapes only, and immediately immersed in a disinfectant solution, or, if disposable, placed in a closed container. Once a mask has been worn, it is a source of infection and under no circumstances must it be kept for further use.

4. Gowns

Individual gowns which are worn by the nurse while attending to the infant are hung in the area occupied by the infant. The outside of the gown, i.e. the side in contact with the infant, must be clearly marked or indicated by the method of hanging. An adequate supply of gowns is essential, so that daily or if necessary more frequent changes can be carried out.

5. Overcrowding

The nursery should not be overcrowded; sufficient space must be left between each infant. It is recommended that in a premature or sick baby nursery there should be 50 sq. ft. for each infant (Hospital Building Note 21, H.M.S.O. 1963). It is preferable to use cubicles for individual infants. Proper ventilation should be achieved without lowering the temperature of the room.

Care of Feeding Bottles and Teats

Feeding bottles, teats and milk can be a source of infection. After the feed, the bottle and teat are washed in warm soapy water with a bottle brush and rinsed. The bottle is then immersed in a 1 in 80 solution of sodium hypochlorite (Milton), which is made up once every 24 hours. The teat is also immersed in a 1 in 80 solution of sodium hypochlorite made up in a separate container. Alternatively all articles are autoclaved. Boiling as a means of sterilising is not recommended. If it is the only means available, it is essential to ensure that the bottle is filled with water and fully immersed for adequate sterilisation to take place. The bottles and teats are boiled for five minutes.

Preparation of Feeds

Aseptic technique is essential. The feeds are best prepared in a special milk kitchen or, if that is not available, one nurse should be assigned to this duty. Masks and gowns are worn, and windows and doors kept closed. The hands are washed before preparing feeds. Feeding instruction charts are available so that an accurate formula is prepared. When the bottle is filled, the teat is applied by touching only the neck of the teat. The teat is then covered with a sterile bag to prevent contamination while carrying the feed to the infant. Terminal sterilisation may be carried out and is achieved by autoclaving the bottled feeds. Feeds for 24 hours may be prepared and stored in a refrigerator.

Visitors

No visitors should be allowed to enter the premature nursery, but a window should be provided so that parents can see their infants.

Observing Signs of Infection occurring in Infants

Every nurse must be vigilant and report the slightest change from normal in the infant. These include:

ANOREXIA: Refusal of feeds should always be taken as a warning signal of infection and the fact reported immediately.

RISE OR FALL IN BODY TEMPERATURE: A rise and fall in temperature is usually an indication that infection has occurred, but in cases where primary atelectasis is present, i.e. failure of the lung to expand, the temperature tends to be low. Here respirations are rapid, shallow and irregular.

CYANOSIS: This may be due to potassium depletion where diarrhoea is present, or it may indicate a general lack of oxygen, either due to obstruction in the air passages or to atelectasis.

RESPIRATORY DISTRESS: Atelectasis and acute descending infection of the respiratory tract may be the cause.

JAUNDICE: In the premature infant it may be due to:

(a) Immaturity of the liver or the presence of a greater number of fragile immature cells.
(b) Haemolytic disease.
(c) Infection.

URINARY OUTPUT: It may be scanty or abnormally large. The colour, odour or any abnormality in the urine should be noted. Should anything abnormal be observed, a specimen of urine should be obtained, stating clearly the name of the infant and the time the urine was obtained. The doctor should then be notified so that the urine can be tested as soon as possible. Generally urine tests are carried out once per week. Urinary abnormality may be due to:

1. Impairment of renal function; i.e.
   (a) Low glomerular filtration rate.
   (b) Inability to concentrate urine.
   (c) Low clearance of chlorides and urea.
2. Infection

STOOLS: These should change from dark green of meconium to yellow, but the stools remain soft and unformed. Abnormal stools include: Undigested, loose, green stools, the presence of blood either altered or fresh and presence of mucus.

THE INFANT'S MOUTH: This must be examined at each feeding time, i.e. before giving a feed, to determine at the earliest possible moment the presence of white patches on the tongue, gums and buccal mucosa, indicating oral thrush.

SKIN INFECTION: Infection of the nail-bed occurs frequently. Small vesicles present around the umbilicus particularly, and affection of the napkin area may indicate staphylococcal infection.

EYES: Eyes are readily infected and any signs of stickiness of the eyelids should be reported immediately. Smears should be taken for culture.

NASAL DISCHARGE: This should be treated as serious due to danger of spread to the lungs and ears.

EARS: Infection may spread from the nose via the Eustachian tubes to the ears. Fretfulness as well as pyrexia may be indications of infection of the ears and must be reported.

Any infected baby is isolated immediately. The infant requires careful constant supervision, scrupulous cleanliness and minimal handling.

Handling

The more premature the infant, the less handling is advisable. Handling of feeble infants readily precipitates respiratory distress. The infant should be left in the incubator for all nursing procedures until the rectal temperature is stabilised between 36·1-37·2°C or 97-99°F and no colour changes occur. The positioning of the infant varies, but it may be considered desirable to turn the infant on his right side during and after a feed and to the left side midway between the feeds. This is to allow equal expansion of both lungs. Weighing, bathing and feeding are carried out in the incubator. Handling the infant through the apertures is not always easy, particularly when changing the infant's napkin. The following method for changing the napkin may be of help.

The infant's napkin is changed from the opposite side from that used for feeding. He is turned gently to the other side and the soiled napkin is rolled towards the centre and is replaced with a clean one. The area is cleansed either with soap and water or with hexachlorophane skin cleanser which is washed off with water and then dried. The infant is then turned on to the clean napkin. The soiled napkin is removed and the clean one straightened out.

Taking of Temperature

Each infant must have his own thermometer which should be of the low-registering variety. The thermometer may be kept in a solution of disinfectant, or may be kept dry in individual containers. Temperatures should be taken rectally and to prevent disturbing the infant too often, it should coincide with the napkin changes. If the thermometer is kept in a solution of disinfectant it should be rinsed in cool water and lubricated lightly before use. The bulbous end is inserted gently for about 1 inch ($2\frac{1}{2}$ cm.) into the rectum. On withdrawing the thermometer, it is wiped, read, and then washed with plain water or hexachlorophane before replacing it in the container.

Weighing

Provided the infant feeds well and has normal bowel movements, daily weighing is not necessary. Individual scales are ideal and communal ones to be avoided. Babies in incubators can be weighed lying in a canvas sling, suspended from a portable spring balance. If individual scales are not available, bigger infants may be weighed wrapped in their own blankets to avoid exposure, on scales brought to the cot on a trolley. The weight of the blanket can then be subtracted from the total weight. The pan of the scales is covered with a large sheet of paper, a new sheet being used for each baby. The used paper is discarded into a covered container.

Bathing

There is no universal method. Some hospitals advocate bathing with soap and water, oiling, or using hexachlorophane, while others advocate no bathing procedure.

The principal aims are to avoid:
  (*a*) Loss of body heat.
  (*b*) Excessive handling.
  (*c*) Prevention of infection.

OILING

If oiling is the choice, sterile liquid paraffin is used. This is particularly useful when removing blood and vernix.

SOAP AND WATER

Babies weighing 2 kilos or 4 lb. or more may be given a water bath. This may be done occasionally or regularly every second or third day. The temperature of the bath should be 37·8-40°C or 100-104°F. Exposure to cold must be avoided and the infant covered in a warm dry towel. Communal baths are best avoided and either individual fixed basins or bowls used. It is essential to clean the basins or bowls thoroughly after bathing the baby.

HEXACHLOROPHANE

The baby's body is cleansed gently every second day with hexachlorophane skin cleanser. This is washed off with warm tap water. Some units use sterile water. This method is also used to cleanse the buttocks when napkins are soiled.

Care of the Eyes

The eyes should be inspected daily, but routine cleansing is inadvisable. If the eyes are 'sticky' or discharging, a swab is taken to identify the organisms responsible for the infection. Should cleansing be required, warm sterile water or half-strength normal saline and sterile cotton wool may be used on closed eyelids. The swab is held lightly on the eyelids and swabbing should be from the inner to the outer aspect of the eye, using each swab once only.

Care of the Nostrils

If the nostrils are clean, they should not be touched, but the outer nares may be cleaned with sterile cotton wool wrung out in sterile water. If the nostrils require cleaning, a small piece of cotton wool should be rolled and gently inserted into each nostril, using a clean piece of cotton wool for each nostril.

Care of the Ears

If the ears are clean, they should not be touched, but the external part of the ear may require cleaning. This should be done by using a small piece of cotton wool moistened with water. Care must be taken to dry the pinna of the ear and ensure that the area behind the ear is dry. The latter part in particular often becomes red and excoriation readily occurs. The external auditory meatus should not be touched except when specific local treatment is necessary. (For treatment of the ear see Chapter X.)

Care of the Cord

The cord of a premature infant takes longer to separate. It must be kept dry and free from contamination by urine. Covering is not necessary, but the cord and the umbilical area may be treated with methylated spirit. No talcum powder should be used, as this may be a source of infection, but sterile cord powders are available, if necessary.

Feeding of Premature Infants

The method of feeding depends on the ability of the infant to suck and swallow. Most premature infants are able to suck from a bottle, provided a soft teat with a large enough hole is used.

Where possible, breast milk should be given, but since it is expressed, contamination may have occurred. It is therefore pasteurised before it is given to the infant. If breast milk is not available, a dried milk food is used instead.

Small feeding bottles holding 4 ounces (120 ml.) can be used and the teat must contain a hole which will allow an easy flow of milk; i.e. allow the escape of large drops of milk but not a steady stream of milk when inverted. Small feeds of approximately 2 fl. drachms (8 ml.) given every three hours to begin with, after an initial period of starvation from 12-24 hours. These feeds are increased as indicated by the infant's ability and eagerness to take it.

Infants who are unable to suck should be tube fed. Feeding by means of pipette, Belcroy feeder, or spoon carries a great risk of inhalation. When tube feeding, a naso-gastric polyvinyl tube is used which is left in position for five days. Passing a catheter nasally repeatedly at each feed is not recommended because of the danger of trauma to the nasal airway. The nurse must be constantly aware of the risk of aspiration pneumonia due to aspiration of feeds and stomach contents into the lungs causing an inflammatory reaction. To ensure that the tube is in the correct position and patent, the tube can be aspirated.

Technique of Bottle Feeding

Test the temperature of the feed on the back of the hand first. The infant's chest is raised with the left hand and the teat inserted into the mouth. It is important to ensure that the teat is on top of the tongue, since in premature infants the tongue often sticks to the roof of the mouth. The teat must be full of milk so that swallowing of air is avoided. Any air swallowed is brought up by gently rubbing the infant's back. This should be done during and after the feed. The chest and head can be raised for 15 minutes after the feed has been given and the back of the throat inspected to make sure that all the feed has been swallowed. Too much handling of the infant after feeding must be avoided to prevent regurgitation of feeds. Accurate feeding charts should be kept. These will show the amount offered and taken and any remarks made regarding the infant's ability to feed.

Preparation for Dismissal

Infants are usually allowed to go home when their weight is 2-2·5 kg. or 5 or 5½ lb., but before discharge, they should be acclimatised to normal conditions. As the body temperature level rises to normal, the heating of the incubator or cot may be reduced, and as the temperature of the environment is reduced, the infant is gradually dressed, if previously nursed without clothing. If he has been nursed in an incubator, he is transferred to a cot. Handling of the infant is increased, but he must still be protected from draughts and excessive heat loss. Where possible, isolation from other infants should be maintained. Before discharge from hospital the infant should be placed in an environment where the temperature is similar to the one at his home.

The mother is notified of the infant's impending discharge from the hospital and arrangements are made to educate the mother. If at all possible, the mother should be admitted for several days before discharge or, if that is not possible, she should be asked to come daily to the hospital where demonstrations are given of bathing, handling, dressing, preparation and giving of feeds. She must be able to carry out all the above under supervision and must be reasonably confident in handling her child.

The hospital medical social worker is notified of the child's impending discharge from the hospital and contact made with the health visitor of the area, so that inspection of the home prior to discharge and later visits and guidance are available.

Arrangements should be made for the infant to attend the child welfare clinic, where regular weighing and examination can take place. Transport other than public transport should be provided where private arrangements cannot be made, so that the infant is not exposed to direct infection immediately he leaves the hospital.

BIBLIOGRAPHY

Crosse, V. M. (1966). *The Premature Baby*, 6th ed. London: Churchill.

Grulee, G. E. & Eley, R. C. (1952). *The Child in Health and Disease*, 2nd ed. Baltimore: Williams & Wilkins.

Hutchison, J. H. (1967). *Practical Paedriatic Problems*. London: Lloyd Luke.

Kessel, I. (1967). *The Essentials of Paediatrics for Nurses*, 3rd ed. Edinburgh: Livingstone.

Mann, T. P. (1963). Hypothermia in the newborn. *Nurs. Times*, **59**, 15.

Marlow, D. (1965). *Textbook of Paediatric Nursing*, 2nd ed. Philadelphia: Saunders.

Von Sedon, G. (1963). Care of premature babies in Sweden. *Nurs. Mirror*, **115**, 455.

Silver, H. K., Kempe, C. H. & Bruyn, H. B. (1967). *Handbook of Paediatrics*, 7th ed. California: Lange.

CHAPTER V

PRE- AND POST-OPERATIVE NURSING CARE

Up to 1 year; 1-4 years; 4-12 years; emergency operation; immediate post-operative period.

PRE-OPERATIVE CARE OF THE INFANT AND CHILD

THE preparation of the child varies with the degree of illness, with the operation to be undergone, and with age.

Generalised care only will be outlined, but the needs of the child will be considered in the following age groups: (1) newborn to 1 year, (2) 1 year to 4 years, and (3) 4 years to 12 years. As part of the general pre-operative preparation for all age-groups, it is important that a specimen of urine is obtained to test for sugar and albumen. When the child is admitted as an emergency, the first specimen which he passes after admission must be saved and tested.

Care of the Child up to 1 year of age

1. COMFORT, WARMTH AND GENTLE HANDLING are essential to minimise the risk of shock in the ill child. All specific pre-operative procedures should be completed an hour prior to operation to avoid unnecessary exposure. Maintenance of body temperature is important, but excessive heat causing loss of fluid through sweating is harmful.

2. CLEANLINESS. A bath is the normal routine. The site for operation must be cleansed thoroughly and the use of talcum powder avoided. This is not easily removed and has been thought to have been introduced into wounds, causing the formation of adhesions.

Nostrils require careful cleansing. Any hard crust must be softened and removed. This can be done by gently dabbing the crusts with a solution of sodium bicarbonate, normal saline, or water. Crusts, by obstructing the airway, cause secretions to accumulate in the post-nasal passage. Once the crust is loosened, the secretions trickle down to the larynx causing a considerable hazard should this occur during anaesthesia. There is also the possibility that the crust itself may be inhaled.

3. CLOTHING. The infant is dressed in warm, loose clothes with adequate covering for feet and hands. Blankets must not restrict respirations, but should be lightly and loosely covering the infant.

4. HYDRATION. If the operation is elective and the infant healthy, the feeding regime need not be changed until the day of operation when 5 per cent dextrose or dilute sweetened orange juice for the older infant is given at least three hours prior to the time of operation. For the young infant, the 6 a.m. feed may be given at midnight. Thereafter, sweetened fluid four hours before operation.

The ill infant requires careful assessment of fluid and electrolyte balance. Fluid and salt loss if excessive are always replaced prior to operation. Medical orders have to be carried out with great accuracy. Careful observation by the nurse and reporting of any change in the condition of the infant is essential. Dramatic changes may take place with little warning, but more often are insidious in onset and, therefore, more difficult to determine. This requires skilled appreciation of the infant's condition and accurate assessment of fluid lost is of the utmost importance. It is here the nurse has a vital role to play.

5. BLADDER AND BOWEL. The nurse taking the infant to the operating theatre should know when the child last passed urine and had a bowel movement. Bowel washouts are never given as a routine but may be necessary for specific operations.

6. PREMEDICATION. This is ordered by the anaesthetist and is generally given by a member of the nursing staff. Depressant drugs are best avoided in infants. It is important for the infant to be awake and crying immediately after completion of an anaesthetic. This is to ensure that he will expand his lungs fully and that the cough and swallowing reflexes are present, thus avoiding the risk of aspiration of vomitus.

Atropine sulphate is given to depress salivary and bronchial secretions. It does not sedate the child in any way.

7. IDENTIFICATION. It is essential that all infants undergoing operation should have identification bracelets, giving name, age, ward and hospital number. Case notes, charts, and X-ray plates are taken to theatre with the child, but these are not proof of identity. The nurse accompanying the child must be confident

that she has the correct child, that she knows his name, age, and diagnosis, and that all pre-operative care has been carried out. The weight of the child is also important for calculating the dose of relaxant drug which may be given by the anaesthetist. The weight should be written where it can be easily found.

Pre-operative Care 1 to 4 years

1. COMFORT. In this age-group, the child cannot understand what is about to happen. Everything is strange and unless the child has been in hospital for some time and knows the nurses, he feels insecure and resentful of all around him. The presence of his mother until he is asleep and under the influence of the sedative will help such a child. If this is not possible, suitable distractions, such as positioning the bed at a window and avoiding the tantalising sight of the breakfast trolley, will help. Warmth and careful handling must be considered as for the infant.

2. CLEANLINESS, including care of the nostrils, as for the infant.

3. CLOTHING. Clothing needs to be loose fitting, preferably tying down the back. Turkish towelling is a suitable material for gowns as it can be boiled; it is also warm and does not cause fluff in the theatre. The ties of the gown should be loosened while in the anaesthetic room, and the gown then slipped off in theatre without any disturbance.

4. HYDRATION. Normally, a glucose drink three to four hours prior to operation is given. Dehydration, if present, is corrected as ordered by the medical staff prior to operation. Careful observation of the child and reporting of excessive fluid loss is essential— see similar paragraph relative to the infant.

5. BLADDER AND BOWEL. No specific care is given to the bowel, other than to ensure that the child is not unduly constipated. Routine purging is unnecessary and dangerous. It can also cause dehydration and exhaustion; it also leads to constipation in the post-operative period.

The child who is toilet trained should be encouraged to use his 'potty'. A child going to theatre with a full bladder may void while induction of anaesthesia is taking place. Should it remain unobserved, a full bladder could cause some difficulty to the surgeon if an abdominal operation were being performed. The nurse taking the child to theatre must know when the child last passed urine.

6. PREMEDICATION. This is dependent on the age and the condition of the child, also the type of anaesthesia which is to be given. From approximately one and a half years upwards, some preoperative sedation may be ordered. It is essential that this is given an adequate period beforehand, usually a minimum of one hour, to allow the child to settle and sleep. Atropine sulphate, or alternative drug, is given to diminish bronchial secretions and saliva. This is given by subcutaneous injection thirty minutes prior to operation. These drugs must be clearly written on the anaesthetic record, and the time at which they were given entered.

7. IDENTIFICATION AND TRANSFER TO THEATRE. Identity bracelets are applied to all children regardless of age-group, and are a wise safety precaution. If bracelets are not provided, adhesive tape with the same particulars firmly attached to the wrist is necessary to ensure that the correct patient is operated upon. It is essential that the nurse accompanying the child knows him well and can give him the comfort and reassurance he needs should he rouse on the way to the operating theatre. She must also know all the necessary particulars, as outlined for the infant. A child who has had a sedative is drowsy and may even be disorientated. He should, therefore, never be left on a trolley unguarded for even a moment.

Care of the Child 4 years to 12 years

1. COMFORT. The older child requires to have some brief but simple explanation. He should be warm, comfortable, free from fear, and, when he reaches the theatre, should be asleep or in a sleepy state. The child should know and trust the nurse who accompanies him. A frightened child, not properly prepared, is much more likely to suffer from post-operative vomiting and the hazards this entails. His recovery will be more prolonged and less pleasant. Fear increases the basal metabolic rate and the oxygen requirement of the body.

Preparation aims at sending the child to theatre as fit as possible, both mentally and physically, and to achieve this, wise planning is essential. Expert guidance given by the ward sister is important, as the needs of individual children vary so much. Adequate, but not excessive warmth and careful handling are important whatever the age-group.

2. CLEANLINESS as for the infant is equally important for all age-groups.

3. CLOTHING. As for the younger child.

4. HYDRATION. Fluids given on the morning of operation should be sweetened. One cup of tea, or a glucose drink, three to four hours prior to operation is normally adequate. If dehydration is present, this must be corrected and medical orders carried out with care.

5. BLADDER AND BOWEL. Occasionally the older child may be reluctant to use a urinal or bedpan, and, if possible, he should be allowed up to the toilet. It is important to ensure that he passes urine before premedication is given and not disturbed after he has been left to sleep.

Bowel care as for the younger child.

6. PREMEDICATION. As for the younger child. When sedation is given, correct timing is important. If given too early, or too late, the child is non-cooperative; also when given too late, recovery is slow and respirations depressed.

7. IDENTIFICATION AND TRANSFER. As for the younger child.

PREPARATION FOR EMERGENCY OPERATION

In addition to the points already mentioned, it is essential to discover when the child last ate, or was given fluids. It is said that the stomach will empty within three hours after a three-course meal. Shock, or fright, will, however, delay this emptying and it is, therefore, important to know the time of the accident in relation to the taking of food. In such circumstances, foodstuffs have been found in the stomach twelve to twenty-four hours after a meal.

A child going to the operating theatre four hours after taking a meal cannot, therefore, be presumed to have a stomach empty of all food content if the accident occurred one hour after taking a meal. If in any doubt at all, a large stomach tube—size 21 F.G. or 12 E.G. for a small child, size 24 F.G. or 14 E.G. for eight years and upwards—should be passed and a gastric lavage given. The child may vomit when the tube is passed. This is perhaps the best way of ensuring that all food has been removed. If any doubt exists, the operation should be delayed. The anaesthetist should be informed of all measures carried out and the possibility of foodstuff being retained.

For the ill child with an intestinal obstruction, an oesophageal tube No. 11-14 F.G. or 6-8 E.G., is passed, or No. 9 F.G. or 4 E.G. for the infant in the neo-natal period. This is aspirated by syringe and the tube is left open, or attached to the suction apparatus at 5 in. Hg or 12 cm. Hg vacuum. Such tubes should never be clamped off. It is an escape for gas as well as for fluid. There is a great danger that the ill or weak infant may inhale vomitus, also respiratory distress can become acute if there is abdominal distension. These can be avoided if the stomach is kept empty and the tube is open.

It is important that the anxiety of the older child should not be increased by unnecessary agitation around him. Whenever possible, he should be given adequate time to settle down and sleep prior to the operation.

Since hyperpyrexia may lead to febrile convulsions during anaesthesia, the anaesthetist must be notified of it in advance. In hyperpyrexia, there is a high tissue demand for oxygen leading to a rapid respiratory rate which is extremely exhausting. The respirations are shallow and there is no full expansion of the lungs. This may be partly due to anxiety and can be relieved by adequate sedation. Tepid sponging may be carried out to reduce the body temperature.

CARE OF THE CHILD IN THE IMMEDIATE POST-OPERATIVE PERIOD

The essential need is for the nurse to recognise the early signs of respiratory obstruction, and appreciate immediately any change in the child's general condition. She must be able to act calmly, quickly and confidently in an emergency. This can only be if she has learned to observe properly and understands the dangers and difficulties which may arise.

Points of Importance with Children of all Age-groups

1. Careful handling.
2. Maintenance of a clear airway.
3. Maintenance of correct body temperature.
4. Maintenance of correct fluid and electrolyte balance.
5. Adequate sedation.

CAREFUL HANDLING. Great care must be taken when transferring a child from the operating table to trolley or cot. Careless lifting or positioning may well cause respiratory embarrassment

D

due to the tongue, or secretions, partially obstructing the airway and resulting in laryngeal spasm. Two nurses are required and three are necessary for the older child. One nurse supports the child's head, keeping it low and keeping the neck in correct alignment. The lifting movement must not begin until everyone is ready. The head of the trolley should be placed at the foot of the table so that awkward movements are avoided (Fig. 8). It is also

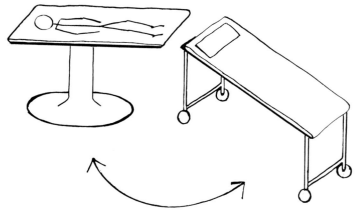

Fig. 8
Position of trolley in relation to the operating table

important to remember that the eyes could readily sustain an injury when the reflex mechanism is depressed and the eyelids are open.

MAINTENANCE OF A CLEAR AIRWAY. It is usual for the child to be transferred from the operating theatre to his own bed in a recovery room or to a position in the ward where resuscitation equipment is immediately available. For equipment and use of suction see Chapter XX.

To ensure that the airway is kept clear, it is essential that the nurse watches the child and listens to his breathing very carefully until the cough reflex has returned and the child has been fully awake. The sound of air being drawn through secretions at the back of the throat, stridor or laboured breathing are indications for instant action. If correct positioning of the child and an attempt to clear the airway make no improvement, the anaesthetist must be sent for without delay.

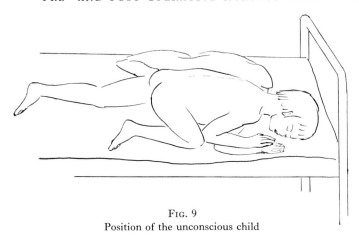

FIG. 9
Position of the unconscious child

Laboured breathing may be very obvious with exaggerated chest movements, or it may develop more insidiously with an indrawing of the lower ribs and at the neck above the manubrium sterni as accessory muscles of respiration come into play.

The position of maximum safety which enables secretions or vomitus to be cleared from the mouth and is least likely to cause inhalation of such, is the lateral position as in Figures 9 and 10.

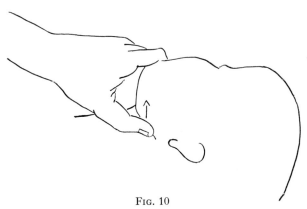

FIG. 10
Method of holding jaw when the child is vomiting. Head is turned to the side. The thumb is on the angle of the jaw pressing forward.

The lower shoulder must not be tucked underneath the body because of the danger of pressure with resultant damage to the
brachial nerve. If the child must be nursed on his back, the head
should be extended and the chin supported as in Figure 11.

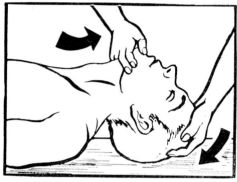

FIG. 11
Method of supporting the jaw when the child is on
his back, to obtain maximum airway. (Reprinted
by kind permission of Smith & Nephew Ltd.)

It is safe to leave the child only when he has been fully awake
and his general condition gives no cause for anxiety. He may then
be made comfortable and allowed to settle to sleep. The infant
should be encouraged to give a cry to ensure good expansion of
his lungs.

MAINTENANCE OF CORRECT BODY TEMPERATURE. It is important
to prevent heat loss and maintain the normal body temperature.
Overheating is also harmful as it increases the basal metabolic
rate and consequently oxygen requirement. The child should be
returned to a warmed cot but artificial means of heat removed
unless very stringent safety precautions are taken. The risk of
burning an unconscious patient due to the absence of any reflex
action is very real. It is also important to ensure that the room
temperature is adequate, a minimum temperature of 18·3°C or
65°F being advised. Heavy bed clothes should never be used in
an attempt to give warmth as these restrict chest movement and
embarrass respiration.

The use of an incubator is ideal for the infant still in the neonatal period. The temperature and humidity can be kept constant and there is no need for clothing.

A sudden rise or fall in body temperature, occurring in the post-operative period, can be detrimental to the child and must be reported to the surgeon whose instructions are then carried out with care.

For accurate recording of the temperature, it is essential that it be taken the same way on each occasion. If it is requested that a rectal recording should be taken, this will be up to 0·5°C and from 1-2°F higher than a skin temperature. The thermometer must be inserted 1-1½ inches into the rectum and the buttocks lightly compressed to get an accurate reading.

FLUID AND ELECTROLYTE BALANCE. Children recover very quickly from anaesthesia and may crave a drink soon after their return to the ward. The time when they can be given oral fluids depends on the nature of the operation and the condition of the child. It may well be that they can safely be given a few sips of water followed two or three hours later by a glucose drink, and on the evening of operation a very light meal. Should vomiting occur, fluids are discontinued temporarily until the child has settled.

The infant, if he has undergone a minor operation, may be given a half-strength milk feed or glucose water approximately three hours after operation. Thereafter normal feeds can be resumed and any appropriate solid diet given the next day.

The restoration of correct fluid and electrolyte balance in such circumstances is a simple matter. The child will demand his fluids and usually tolerates them well.

Post-anaesthetic vomiting is not usual, though it may be marked in a child who was very emotionally upset and frightened prior to operation. If it persists, it must be reported, the amount and frequency being carefully recorded. Comfort and reassurance with adequate sedation are important factors. Opiates are best avoided as they may produce vomiting.

The importance of having a nurse known to the child and one he has confidence in helps tremendously at this time. Parents can contribute greatly to soothing and calming the anxious child provided they themselves are able to control their own anxiety.

The maintenance of fluid and electrolyte balance of the ill child requires skill and knowledge of the needs of the child. The nurse has a vital part to play.

Meticulous observations and reporting of the slightest change in the condition of the child is essential. An infant may give little cause for anxiety yet within one hour his condition can deteriorate appreciably. The ability to see this change at the earliest moment, to understand the significance and summon a medical opinion is important.

Medical orders require to be carried out carefully and at the appropriate times. Assessment of fluid intake and fluid loss must be accurate and recordings must be clearly and carefully entered on the fluid balance chart. All forms of fluid loss should be considered though not all can be measured. Care must be taken not to cause excessive fluid loss through perspiration.

SEDATION. It is unwise and unkind to leave a child of any age-group without sedation should he be restless, distressed, or complaining of pain. In such instances, the child should be made as comfortable as possible and doctor's orders sought as to the type and amount of sedation required.

Pain and restlessness quickly exhaust a child, oxygen demand is greater and blood pressure may reach a dangerously low level should these symptoms be allowed to persist.

BIBLIOGRAPHY

Brunner, L. S., Emerson, C. P. Jnr., Ferguson, L. K., Suddarth, D. S. (1964). *Textbook of Medical-Surgical Nursing.* Philadelphia: Lippincott.
Dennison, W. M. (1968). *Surgery in Infancy and Childhood,* 2nd ed. Edinburgh: Livingstone.
Mason Brown, J. J. (1962). *Surgery of Childhood.* London: Arnold.
Oppé, T. E. (1961). *Modern Textbook of Paediatrics for Nurses.* London: Heinemann.
Wilkinson, A. W. (1968). *Body Fluids in Surgery,* 3rd ed. Edinburgh: Livingstone.

CHAPTER VI

WARD DRESSINGS

Principles; specific techniques; removal of sutures; corset dressing; watershed dressing; Elastoplast; Netalast; peritoneal drainage tubes; finger dressing.

GAINING THE CHILD'S CONFIDENCE

THE importance of gaining the child's confidence when dressings have to be changed is an essential part of the technique. A wound is much more likely to become contaminated when a child is crying and will not keep still. The procedure will also take much longer and the upset caused is not likely to be readily forgotten, making subsequent dressings no easier to perform. This state of affairs arises through a natural fear of being hurt. Several points must, therefore, be considered when carrying out dressings in a children's ward.

Trust

The child who has trust in the nurse about to perform the dressing is much more likely to accept what is in store for him. Truthfulness is essential. It is pointless to say that something will not be painful when it will; this is the first way to destroy trust.

Distraction

A nurse who can keep a child's attention diverted with a story or a toy will contribute greatly to maintaining a calm atmosphere. The approach to each child varies. Some are intensely interested in what is happening and like to see everything; for others, it is much wiser to keep instruments out of sight and distract attention from the proceedings.

Good Technique

It is important to study what causes the child pain or discomfort and endeavour to find some means of avoiding it. Very few dressings which are carried out in the ward, need cause pain and a nurse should constantly be striving to improve her technique. It is not wise to persist in changing dressings if undue pain is being caused, or if the child is very distressed. In such circumstances, suitable sedation may be given and once the child is calm the procedure will be carried out more readily.

Observation

Assessment of the condition of the wound and the progress of healing must be made so that an accurate report may be given to the surgeon.

Reward

This is very important to a child and praise should be given where it is due. The sweet box should not be long in appearing after dressing time. This does not mean that the child who has been upset should be made to feel bad. Only encouragement and understanding will allay fear, and fear is the factor which causes most distress.

THE USE OF A TREATMENT ROOM. This does reduce the amount of tension in a ward at dressing time. Whether or not it reduces the risk of cross infection is a matter of debate. A treatment room with air conditioning which creates a complete change of air every 10 minutes is recommended (Hospital Building Note). When it is necessary to use the ward, it is important to reduce traffic to the minimum and all cleaning, dusting, and bed making should be completed one hour before dressings commence.

Adaptation of methods to suit circumstances and available equipment is necessary, but whatever method is used, certain guiding principles must be observed. Techniques should be based on the current findings of research in an effort to control the risk of cross infection.

GUIDING PRINCIPLES IN DRESSING TECHNIQUES

1. **The Hands** can only be rendered surgically clean and are not sterile. They must, therefore, not come into direct contact with a wound or dressing. Wet hands are liable to cause contamination, therefore hands should be washed carefully and dried on a clean towel.

2. **Gloves.** It may be considered necessary on occasion to use hands rather than forceps for a particular part of the dressing. In these circumstances, sterile gloves should be worn and discarded after that dressing. The mere washing of gloves does not render them sterile.

3. **Masks** are not advocated by everyone, though most surgeons recommend their use when dressing open wounds. They are a danger if not used properly (Chapter III). When in use, all care must be taken to ensure that they remain an adequate barrier. They should never be fingered and disposable ones should be renewed at the appropriate time.

4. **Gowns** may be worn when carrying out a dressing for an infected wound. The gown must be discarded on completion of the dressing. Alternatively, a disposable apron may be used.

5. **Exposure.** The atmosphere is not sterile and therefore any wound exposed to it may become contaminated. Similarly articles which come into contact with the wound, if exposed to the atmosphere, may also lead to contamination. The wound should, therefore, be exposed for as short a time as possible and all articles for use must be kept covered.

6. **Equipment.** Dressing trolleys should be of simple design, easily cleaned, with large 4-in. wheels for ease of movement.

Composite packs containing instruments, dressings and containers are to be preferred to a system whereby several packs may have to be opened for one dressing. Completely disposable packs can be obtained, but the quality of instruments is as yet not always acceptable for specialised work.

Packs must be stored in an area which is free from damp. The shelf life of paper-wrapped sealed packs is said to be indefinite, providing the pack is not torn in any way or has become damp. The atmosphere in the treatment room will at times have a high bacterial count and it is, therefore, unwise to use it for the storage of equipment, sterile or otherwise. The practice of shaking articles out of a bag on to a sterile field is not a good one. Inevitably some dust from the outside of the bag may be shaken on to the area.

Each pack must be carefully checked before use to ensure seals or colour coding is correct and that the exterior wrap is not damaged in any way.

7. **Soiled Dressings.** Individual disposable bags may be at-

tached to the side of the trolley and, as soon as each dressing is completed, the bag is closed and put into a foot-operated bin. The direct use of such a bin is not advocated because of the danger of air pollution each time the bin is opened.

8. **Routine.** A routine for ward dressings should be established with clear guidance as to preparation, execution and disposal of used items. This should be in writing in a ward policy manual. This is an important contributory factor in the elimination of poor technique.

Cheatles' Forceps. Since the discovery that the *Pseudomonas pyocyaneus* and other such organisms can flourish in disinfectants used in receptacles in the ward, the Cheatles' Forceps has been regarded as a dangerous object. Should it be required for setting such detailed procedures as cardiac catheterisation, the forceps should be in individual packs, autoclaved, and used for setting one procedure only.

Drums. It is widely accepted that the individual pack is to be preferred to the drum, or any communal type of container. Exposure of the contents of the drum to the atmosphere on each occasion it was opened led to contamination of contents. Faulty drums with ill fitting lids were not unknown. Where drums are used as individual containers for specialised equipment, it is safer to have the equipment seal-wrapped. As with any articles to be autoclaved, drums should not be packed too tightly, thereby ensuring that all the contents are sterilised.

WARD DRESSINGS

METHOD. Individual packets are used and contain all the necessary articles for the dressing except the lotions, which are poured into the gallipots once the packet is opened (Fig. 12). Requirements as in Figure 12. Gowns are worn for infected wounds.

Two nurses are necessary; the dresser, who prepares the trolley and performs the dressing, and the assistant, who prepares and looks after the child.

The trolley is first washed with soap and water, and dried. Disposable paper towels should be used in preference to a cloth or duster which may be a source of infection.

Both nurses wash and dry their hands on individual towels and put on gowns and masks. The assistant places the child in the correct position and removes the bandages. She then holds the child and distracts his attention.

The dresser proceeds as in Figure 12. The dressing is gently removed from the wound using forceps. Should it be adherent, it may be necessary to soak it with warm saline. The forceps are then discarded. Using forceps, the wound is cleansed and covered with a swab. The surrounding skin is then cleansed, working from the wound outwards. Finally, the area is dried and the appropriate dressings applied. The assistant then covers the dressings with adhesive tape or bandage and makes the child comfortable.

When an assistant is available to pour lotions and produce setting forceps (step O, Fig. 12), the second washing of hands may be omitted and the setting forceps used to remove the dressing prior to them being discarded.

Soiled dressings are sealed in their bag and put into closed containers. Instruments are discarded into a container which is closed or immersed in a disinfectant. Salvage is collected into a bag. Hands are washed and dried, and the articles are cleared away. The trolley is washed thoroughly with soap and water, sprayed with hexachlorophane and allowed to dry.

Clean wounds should always be dressed before infected wounds, as inevitably organisms will escape into the atmosphere, leading to contamination of other wounds.

SOME SPECIFIC TECHNIQUES

Removal of Sutures

The length of time the sutures remain in position is dependent upon the location and tension. It may vary from two to fourteen days. Facial sutures are removed in the shortest possible time to lessen the possibility of a scar.

Requirements as for dressing. In addition 1 pr. fine stitch scissors

A disposable stitch cutter is available which is excellent for use with older children, but it is not recommended if there is a possibility of the child moving suddenly.

Dry surfaces are less likely to become infected and it is for this reason that some surgeons prefer the sutures to be removed from clean wounds without initial cleansing of the skin.

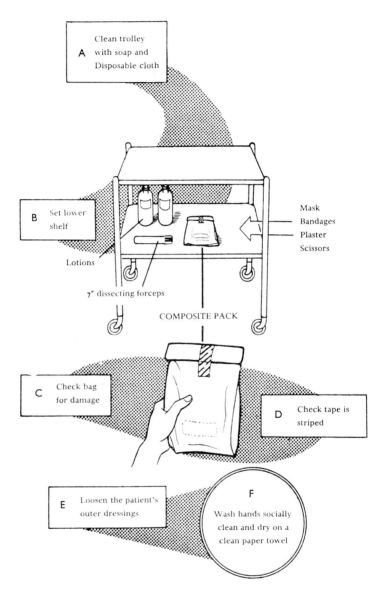

A Clean trolley with soap and Disposable cloth

B Set lower shelf

Mask
Bandages
Plaster
Scissors

Lotions

7" dissecting forceps

COMPOSITE PACK

C Check bag for damage

D Check tape is striped

E Loosen the patient's outer dressings

F Wash hands socially clean and dry on a clean paper towel

FIG. 12A

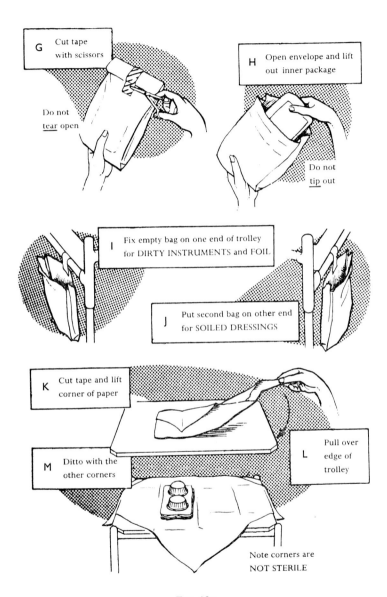

G Cut tape with scissors

Do not tear open

H Open envelope and lift out inner package

Do not tip out

I Fix empty bag on one end of trolley for DIRTY INSTRUMENTS and FOIL

J Put second bag on other end for SOILED DRESSINGS

K Cut tape and lift corner of paper

M Ditto with the other corners

L Pull over edge of trolley

Note corners are NOT STERILE

FIG. 12B

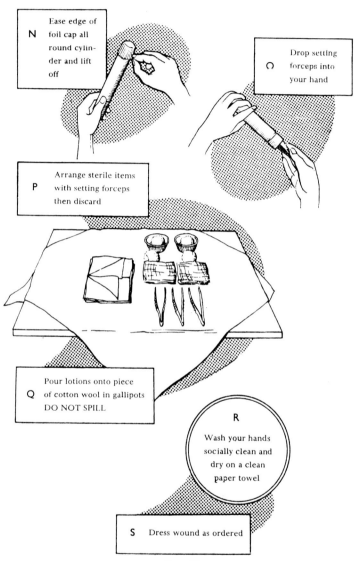

N Ease edge of foil cap all round cylinder and lift off

O Drop setting forceps into your hand

P Arrange sterile items with setting forceps then discard

Q Pour lotions onto piece of cotton wool in gallipots DO NOT SPILL

R Wash your hands socially clean and dry on a clean paper towel

S Dress wound as ordered

Fig. 12c

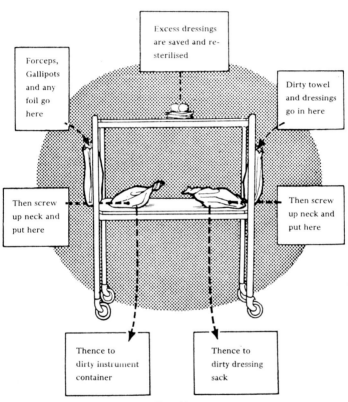

CLEARING UP

Excess dressings are saved and re-sterilised

Forceps, Gallipots and any foil go here

Dirty towel and dressings go in here

Then screw up neck and put here

Then screw up neck and put here

Thence to dirty instrument container

Thence to dirty dressing sack

FIG. 12D

Adapted from basic dressing technique using sterile packs prepared by Bowater-Scott Corporation, Ltd. in conjunction with Guy's Hospital. (Reprinted with kind permission from both.)

The principles to be observed in removing sutures are :

1. Allay the child's fears and have him quiet and relaxed.

2. Any part of the suture which has been exposed on the surface must not be pulled through the underlying tissue.

3. The suture should be cut in one place only to ensure that no part is left under the skin. The exception to this rule is the mattress suture.

The removal of sutures should never be a painful performance unless the sutures have become deeply embedded. It is wise to remove first the one that obviously will not cause pain. This gains the child's confidence and the procedure will be much easier. The knot should never be grasped with the dissecting forceps and lifted up. This causes just enough pain to make him cry out and any movement at this point makes the operation more difficult. The scissors are slipped under the stitch (the blade flat as in Figure 13) and cut where the suture enters the skin. The blade

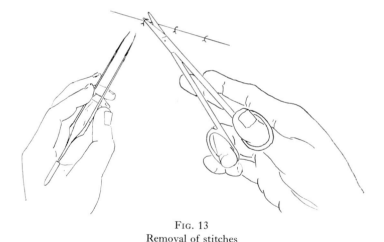

Fig. 13
Removal of stitches

of the scissors is placed on the suture line and the knot is pulled gently with the forceps.

Corset Dressing

This type of dressing may be used when support is required in an effort to unite a wound. It may also be used when frequent dressings are required and a binder is not satisfactory, or when adhesive tape or Elastoplast would have to be reapplied frequently on an abdominal wound. If to give support, the secret of successful application is to bring the Elastoplast from far enough behind to give adequate purchase. The ends of the Elastoplast should be turned over the entire dressing and the eyelets made by cutting holes along the edge. The edges should not meet; approximately one inch space gives an adequate margin for tightening the corset. Narrow tape is threaded through the eyelets. Only the tape needs to be undone when changing the dressing (Fig. 14).

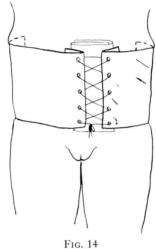

FIG. 14
Corset dressing

Dressings

Wounds heal more quickly if dressing changes do not cause damage to the granulating epithelium and dressings that do not adhere to the wound are less painful to remove. Melolin XA is one type of dressing designed to cause the minimum disturbances to nature's healing process. It is a perforated polyester film on an absorbent dressing and is readily peeled off the wound.

Airstrip dressings (Fig. 15) form a satisfactory covering for a closed wound. They are simple to apply and stay in position well, conform to the suture line, and are water repellent. It has also been observed that these dressings are more easily removed, causing no pain and there is usually no adhesive left on the surrounding skin, thus avoiding the use of methylated ether.

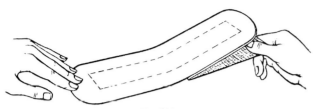

Fig. 15

Airstrip ward dressing demonstrating the method of application. (Reprinted by kind permission of Smith &
Nephew Ltd.)

Watershed Dressing

This type of dressing is useful where there is a closed wound
adjoining a fistula, colostomy, or discharging wound. It is made
of waterproof adhesive tape. Two equal lengths of four-inch
broad strapping are used, a half inch to one inch of the entire
length is turned back and the remaining three to three and a half
inches stuck together. There is now a double length of adhesive
tape with a base to attach to the skin between the wound and the

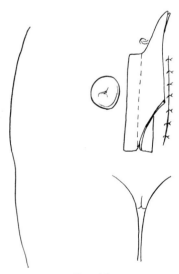

Fig. 16
Watershed dressing

fistula. The wound can then be sealed with an airstrip, or other form of dressing and an absorptive dressing applied to the discharging wound. It is essential that the skin is dry and the adhesive tape applied smoothly with no wrinkles where leakage from the discharging wound could penetrate (Fig. 16).

Use of Elastoplast or Adhesive Tape

Bandages or binders do not always stay in position if a child is ambulant and for this reason Elastoplast is ideal. The removal of Elastoplast is often the most painful part of a dressing and if this has to be done frequently the skin may become very sore. Therefore, when it is known that a dressing will require frequent changing, a piece of Elastoplast covering the surrounding skin, to which the dressing can be attached, will overcome the problem. This need not be changed daily, but only when it becomes soiled. The outer Elastoplast must be cut smaller and if turned in at the end, removal will be much easier (Fig. 17).

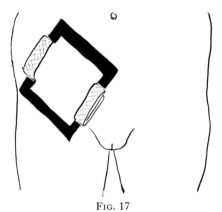

FIG. 17

Technique of fixing dressing to an underlay of adhesive tape, which does not require to be removed each time the dressing is changed.

Removal of Elastoplast. The skin should be eased down from under the adhesive by a swab soaked in methylated ether or solvent. The Elastoplast should never be pulled up from the skin.

Micropore is an adhesive tape which is particularly valuable for use with children. It is much less painful to remove and can be obtained in various widths. It has also been found to cause fewer skin reactions than other types of adhesive.

Netalast

Netalast provides a simple means of keeping a dressing in place in an awkward position. It is light, comfortable and quickly applied.

Shortening of Peritoneal Drainage Tubes

This is not a pleasant task but seldom need be very painful if care is taken. Everything should be in readiness for the dressing; with a large safety pin clamped in a strong pair of artery forceps. The drain is held by dressing forceps and the suture cut; it is then levered gently upwards, usually until it has been removed about one and a half inches, the amount being dependent upon the surgeon's wishes. The decision is based on the length of time he wants the drain to stay in place and this is dependent upon the amount of drainage expected. The drain is held firmly with forceps at the level of insertion through the skin and the safety pin is inserted through the drain just above the forceps. The pin is

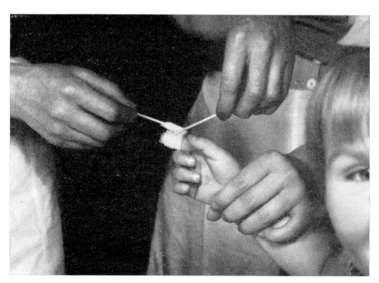

Fig. 18
Finger dressing

then fastened, still using forceps. The excess drain is cut off. The wound is cleaned, dried and the dressings applied. The drain should not be cut until the pin is inserted in case it should slip back into the wound. It is important that the child should not see the safety pin if he is at all apprehensive.

Finger Dressing

The difficulty of trying to maintain a sound technique and produce a good dressing, which will remain in position, is not easy when the part is a tiny finger. The use of applicators wound with ribbon gauze has proved helpful. It also has the additional advantage of being much less frightening to a child than forceps (Fig. 18).

Dressed applicators for cleansing can also be used. These should be prepared beforehand and sterilised, or products such as Johnson and Johnson buds can be used.

BIBLIOGRAPHY

Collins, M. (1967). Complicated dressings made simple. *Nurs. Mirror*, **124**, 13.
Ellison Nash, D. F. (1965). *Principles and Practice of Surgical Nursing*. 3rd ed. London: Arnold.
Fuerst, E. V. & Wolff, L. (1964). *Fundamentals of Nursing*, 3rd ed. Unit 3 Part 8, Unit 15 Part 40 & 41. Philadelphia: Lippincott.
London, P. S. (1967). Wound Dressings. *Nurs. Times*, **63**, 20.
Medical Research Council (1951). *The Control of Cross Infection in Hospitals*. London: H.M.S.O.
Ministry of Health (1964). *Children's Ward*. Hospital Building Note 23. London: H.M.S.O.
Ross, J. S. & Wilson, K. J. W. (1965). *Foundations of Nursing and First Aid*, 4th ed. Edinburgh: Livingstone.

CHAPTER VII

FEEDING PROBLEMS IN THE SURGICAL WARD

Feeding an infant with cleft lip and palate; Pierre-Robin syndrome; maintaining dietary requirements.

THE vast majority of children in surgical wards present no greater feeding problems than are met with elsewhere, nor do they differ greatly from the normal child in this respect. Those, who have some congenital abnormality, sustained injury or undergone surgery, will inevitably have a period of reduced intake, but this is seldom prolonged and any deficit is readily made good in convalescence. When the problem does arise, however, it is of major importance, and there is some degree of urgency in instituting treatment.

ESTABLISHMENT OF FEEDING IN INFANTS WITH CLEFT LIP AND PALATE

The infant with a cleft lip and palate may appear grossly deformed to the mother at first sight. It is, however, very important to reassure her that plastic surgical repair will restore the lip to its natural line and the palate to its natural function.

The establishment of feeding has been made very much easier with the use of an orthodontic splint (Fig. 19). This is a small acrylic plate, which is fitted as soon as possible after birth and kept in night and day. The splint aids in bringing the alveolar margin into alignment thus making the task of repairing the lip easier. It also separates the oral cavity from the nasal cavity, so preventing the passage of fluids into the nasal passages with subsequent deafness due to tissue changes and extension of infection to the middle ear. The splint enables the infant to be fed normally, as the functions of sucking, swallowing and breathing are restored.

The mother does require support and guidance as the establishment of feeding will take longer. Fear and apprehension are all too easily transmitted to an infant and will certainly only contribute to the difficulties if allowed to develop. It is essential to hold the baby confidently and slightly more upright than usual. Support may be necessary for the lower jaw.

The mother can be assured that with diligent use of the splint in early infancy, children do not suffer acute speech disorders and respond well to speech therapy.

The plate is removed after each feed and washed under the running tap using a tooth brush and salt. It is replaced immediately. It is necessary for the splint to be readjusted by the orthodontist every two to three weeks.

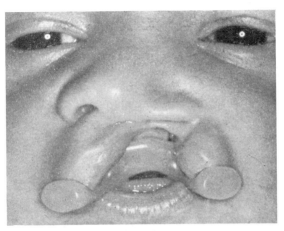

FIG. 19
Orthodontic plate for infant with cleft palate and lip.
(Reprinted from Dennison, W. M., *Surgery in Infancy and Childhood*.)

Weaning can be commenced during this period. The splint is not necessary after the lip is repaired and this usually takes place when the baby is three to four months old.

Without a plate, it is not possible to feed the infant by bottle. Cup and spoon is the simplest method. The important factor is reassuring the mother that the baby is unlikely to choke and that he can get an adequate feed once feeding is established. Patience and perseverence are the greatest attributes. Spluttering is alarming for the mother and upsetting to the baby as well as contributing to middle ear complications already mentioned. Every endeavour should be made to reduce it to the minimum. It is advisable to give only small spoonfuls of milk at a time, to talk to the baby, and try to keep him calm while feeding. A cross baby is very difficult to deal with and for this reason feeding on demand is advocated.

THE PROBLEMS OF THE INFANT WITH PIERRE-ROBIN SYNDROME

An infant born with a cleft palate and retardation of the jaw (mandibular retrognathia) is said to have a Pierre-Robin Syndrome. This presents a considerable challenge to the nursing staff who have to care for the infant. The first few weeks are critical ones for this baby. The dangers are, firstly, of the infant's tongue falling back and blocking the airway; secondly, because there is a failure of development of the suck and swallow mechanism, the infant does not co-ordinate all movements correctly and may swallow when the air passages are not occluded. There is, therefore, grave danger of respiratory obstruction and aspiration pneumonia.

Nursing care is devoted to the prevention of those occurrences.

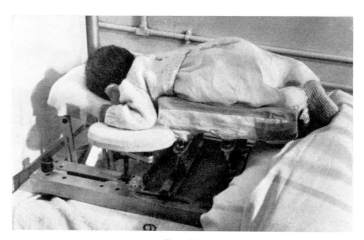

Fig. 20

Frame for infant with Pierre-Robin Syndrome. Note mirror beneath the face to allow easy observation of the jaw and tongue. (Figs. 20 and 21 reprinted by kind permission of the Editor of *Nursing Times* and The Royal Liverpool Children's Hospital.)

1. Position

During the first twenty-four hours, the infant is nursed prone. He requires constant supervision, that is the undivided attention of one nurse. A suction machine with sterile suction catheter should be at the bedside. On any sign of respiratory difficulty, the infant should be picked up, placed in the head-low position, face downwards, and a sharp tap given on the back to bring the tongue forward. Suction should only be used if necessary. Maintenance of the head-low position is not advocated when the infant is in his cot as this tends to cause respiratory embarrassment, especially after feeding.

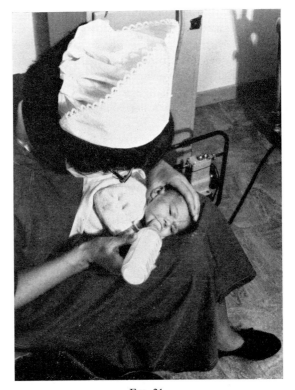

FIG. 21

The feeding position recommended: note sister's left thumb holding the mandible forward; the sucker may be seen in readiness in the background.

To permit the infant to lie prone with face down, a plaster shell on an aluminium frame has been designed (Fig. 20). This is the position of maximum safety and may have to be maintained for two to three months. The jaw does gradually develop and grow forward giving a normal appearance.

2. Feeding

Feeding is commenced after the first twenty-four hours. The ideal to aim for is bottle feeding as this will aid in the development of the jaw. It is, however, a far from easy task requiring great skill and perseverence. A free hand is required to support the jaw, the thumb exerting a forward pressure. The suction machine must be in readiness (Fig. 21). If the infant is becoming exhausted during the establishment of feeding, alternate feeds may be given by the naso-gastric method for a few days. Feeding should commence with approximately 5 ml. sterile water increasing by 5 ml. every four hours until the baby is receiving 30 ml. It is advisable to give the infant sterile water for two to three days and gradually change to milk feeds increasing the amount according to the baby's needs. Water, if inhaled, will be less disastrous than milk.

The type of teat used and the size of hole can only be determined by trial. An ordinary teat with some experimentation in size of the hole is usually satisfactory.

As milk readily enters the naso-pharynx, rhinitis develops and can pose problems when secretions are excessive. Careful cleansing of the nostrils with moist cotton wool should be carried out before and after feeds. Until feeding is established, it is important for these infants to have constant supervision.

MAINTAINING DIETARY REQUIREMENTS

Miss A. B. Sutherland, m.d., f.r.c.s.e.

In considering any child from the standpoint of his or her nutrition, there are four major reasons why feeding difficulty may be encountered.

1. A Prolonged Period of Reduction in Intake

(*a*) Anorexia, from the associated condition, is perhaps the most frequent and important cause of inadequate feeding. Also it is an insidious factor unlikely to be appreciated unless a careful record is kept of what the child is *actually* eating. It is for this reason that in those cases where reduced intake is suspected an accurate recording should be made of *all* intake—weighed and measured if necessary.

(*b*) THE CONDITION ITSELF may be the reason for reduction in intake—for example, a lesion or injury to the face, especially if the region of the mouth is involved, or lesions of the upper gastro-intestinal tract preventing the onward passage of food.

(*c*) TREATMENT OF THE CONDITION may also impose reduction in intake. Here the most frequent cause is repeated procedures under anaesthesia; for example, the frequent change of dressings. The period of starvation which must necessarily accompany the pre- and post-anaesthetic state frequently reduce what would otherwise be a satisfactory intake to unsatisfactory levels. While much improvement is possible by careful control of intake in the late post-anaesthetic period, intake on those days can seldom reach the desired level. Again, this reduction is not appreciated unless accurate intake records are kept.

Such reduction in intake will concern all dietary constituents—protein, calories, vitamins and iron. In addition, because the total intake is low, any protein taken will tend to be used as a calorie source rather than in its normal role of tissue building and replacement.

2. A Period of Excessive Loss Through Increased Secretion

If an unnatural loss of any substance occurs and is not replaced, the only alternative that the body has is to draw on its reserves. Such reserves are in many instances small in amount so that if replacement is not made depletion occurs rapidly.

After any operation or injury, there is a period when the body breaks down its own protein even when an adequate protein intake is provided. The severity and duration of this breakdown depends on the size of the injury, or the operative procedure, ranging from a few days after a simple appendicectomy to as much as three weeks in an extensive burn. In the former, the loss is easily made good in early convalescence; in the latter, it constitutes a severe drain on body reserves.

Another avenue of increased loss is that from a large area of skin loss whether this be the result of skin destruction following an extensive deep burn or from loss of skin and soft tissue consequent upon other injury. In all instances, the loss of exudate from the surface will continue until healing is achieved. Such loss is mainly of protein and salt. (A similar state of affairs will occur in any patient with a continued formation of pus such as occurs in an empyema cavity.)

Increased loss of many substances will occur in intestinal fistulae; the higher the fistula the more severe will it be and depletion will occur rapidly. Similarly, prolonged vomiting from any cause is an important route of increased secretion.

3. A Period of Diminished Absorption

Patients who for any reason have a prolonged period of intestinal injury will lose important constituents in their faeces. A similar state of affairs exists in those who have required extensive resection of the small bowel. In them, there will be failure to absorb almost all constituents of the diet—protein, fat with the fat soluble vitamins, carbohydrate, minerals such as sodium potassium, calcium and iron, the water soluble vitamins, and water.

4. A Period of Increased Requirement

Patients who have had a reduced intake, increased excretion, or diminished absorption, will obviously have an increased requirement of food to make good previous losses, or to keep pace with those that are occurring. In addition, rise in body temperature increases the metabolic rate so that calories are used up faster, and thus continued fever in itself will increase requirement. A more profound rise occurs in the metabolic rate in the extensive burn, greater than that which could be explained by fever.

Thus, there are many reasons for nutrition being inadequate in certain children in surgical wards and the problem in childhood is a more active one because of the smaller reserves and the increased needs of growth and development. In this connection, the normal requirement for healthy children in varying age groups must be known (Table I). Only by making use of such figures is it possible to gauge what the requirement may be, although because the majority of such children are at bed rest, their basic caloric need will not be as high as in the active child. If, for any of these

TABLE I

NORMAL REQUIREMENTS

Age	Protein gm.	Calories	Iron gm.	Calcium gm.	Vit.A I.U.	Vit.D I.U.	Aneurine mg.	Nicotinic Acid mg.	Riboflavine mg.	Vit.C mg.
0 – 1	37	1000	6·5	1·0	3000	800	0·4	4·0	0·6	10·0
1 – 2	40	1150								
2 – 3	45	1300								
3 – 4	45	1400	7·5	1·0	3000	400	0·6	6·0	0·9	15·0
4 – 5	50	1500								
5 – 6	50	1600								
6 – 7	55	1750								
7 – 8	60	1850	10·5	1·0	3000	400	0·8	8·0	1·2	20·0
8 – 9	65	1950								
9 – 10	70	2150								
10 – 11	102	2350								
11 – 14	102	2750	13·5	1·2	3000	400	1·1	11·0	1·6	30·0

Based on the figures of the B.M.A. Committee on Nutrition Report 1950.

reasons outlined above, needs are increased, intake must be in excess of normal requirement.

Provision of the Required Intake

It is unlikely that in such patients an adequate intake can be provided from ward diet, even when the child is encouraged in every possible way. Figure 22 shows the daily intake of a severely

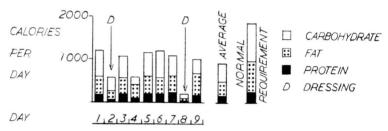

FIG. 22
Intake on ward diet. (Female, aged 7. Burn 50 per cent.)

burned child on ward diet where every effort was made by her nurses to provide a satisfactory intake, and the average daily intake, which is the important factor, is quite inadequate. Such findings are shown repeatedly when accurate intake records are kept. A high protein, high calorie *solid* diet is quite unacceptable to the ill child. In most instances, provision of the intake required for the same child in health will be what is needed. In a few instances, for example, the extensive deep burn, this may have to be increased but in no instance should more than one and a half times the normal protein, or one and one-third times the normal calories be required. Beyond such levels there is a real risk of producing such uncommon syndromes as protein overloading and stress diabetes.

Provision of the required intake is possible in one of two ways:

1. An Oral Fluid Supplement (Table II)

This supplement, in the form of a type of milk shake, is given in addition to solid diet and in the vast majority of patients is all that is required. It provides additional protein and calories in small bulk. It is important that it is given at times which will not interfere with the appetite for the main meals, as these will still provide the greater part of the intake. It is given either in small

TABLE II

SAMPLE OF ORAL SUPPLEMENT

Constituent	Amount gm.	oz.	Protein gm.	Fat gm.	Carbohydrate gm.
Complan (Glaxo)	150	5	46·5	24·0	66·0
Evaporated Milk	180	6	13·7	15·1	22·1
Glucose	15	½	—	—	13·7
Water to	1000	24	—	—	—
Flavouring					
			60·2	39·1	101·8

Volume 1000 ml.
Protein 60 gm.
Calories 1000.
Therefore, each 100 ml. supplies 6·0 g. protein and 100 calories.

quantities of 30 to 60 millilitres (one to two fluid ounces) throughout the waking hours, or in divided portions after the main meals,
during the forenoon or as a bedtime drink. *The requirements for
such a supplement are:*

(i) It must be palatable and capable of variation in flavour.
This is of particular importance where it is required over
long periods of time.

(ii) It must be of suitable consistency.

(iii) It must be simple to prepare so that, if necessary, this can
be done in the ward kitchen.

(iv) It must be of known composition so that its contribution to
the intake can be readily calculated. In the accompanying
formula, the total volume is made up to 1,000 millilitres
(one litre) so that the amounts provided by 100 ml. are
easily calculated, and hence the required volume for any
particular child assessed. This volume must be related to
the age and weight of the child concerned. Young children
will accept up to 300 ml. daily, older children 600 to
800 ml., while the twelve year old will take one litre.

(v) All such supplements should be served ice cold and stored
in a refrigerator. This makes the drink more acceptable
to the child.

2. **Naso-gastric Tube Feeding** (Table III)

This is the method of choice in the following circumstances:

(*a*) Where for local reasons intake by mouth is not possible; for example, severe injuries or lesions of the face and/or mouth.

(*b*) Where the intake of solid food is for varying reasons completely inadequate.

(*c*) Where unconsciousness persists for a period; for example, after a head injury.

(*d*) Where high intakes are required over long periods of time; for example, extensive burns.

(*e*) Where marked depletion is already present.

(*f*) Where it is anticipated that the intake will be inadequate.

Such a method of feeding must be considered before severe nutritional depletion has occurred. Delay in its use until this stage is reached is inevitably associated with failure. If the above indications are observed, this method of feeding should never be used as a last and unavailing resort.

Requirements of the feed:

(i) It should provide the total intake required—this is the purpose of its use, although small amounts of additional solids and of fluids are not contra-indicated.

(ii) It must be of such consistency that it will run easily through the fine bore tube. For practical purposes, it should never be thicker than whole milk. This is not difficult to obtain when the constituents are used in the correct proportions, and remembering also that the day's water requirement must be included.

(iii) The concentration must be kept low, as highly concentrated feeds are seldom well tolerated. Preferably, this concentration should not exceed one calorie per millilitre of feed although up to two calories per millilitre is permissible.

(iv) The total volume must be kept within the limits of acceptance of the individual child and will depend primarily on age.

(v) The formulae should be kept simple so that feeds when necessary can be made up in the ward.

(vi) It is advisable to make up the requirements for a twenty-four-hour period in bulk, all feeds being stored under refrigeration.

(vii) The proportion of fat calories should not exceed 35 per cent of the total.

Administration

1. In most instances, interrupted feeding with the tube left in position is the method of choice. The feed may be given either three- or four-hourly and preferably with a break through the night so that the hours of sleep will be undisturbed; for example, 9 a.m., 12 midday, 3 p.m., 6 p.m., 9 p.m., 12 midnight, and 6 a.m., or 10 a.m., 2 p.m., 6 p.m., 10 p.m., and 6 a.m. Only where tolerance is difficult to achieve, is the continuous method perhaps of some advantage.

2. The individual feed volume will vary with the size and age of the child—200 millilitres in the toddler, 300 millilitres in the young child, and 400 millilitres in the older child. Thus the daily total will be in the order of 1,200 to 2,800 millilitres in the vast majority of instances.

3. Simple gravity drip suffices for delivery of the feed. If the consistency of the feed is correct, no form of pump is required even when using the smallest bore of tube.

4. In commencing tube feeding, it is probably advisable not to start with the full volume which will eventually be required. To build up the volume, give half the final volume initially, increasing this after two to three days to three-quarters, and after a further two to three days including the full volume.

It is most important that children who are being maintained completely by this method should have adequate amounts of all vitamins and iron included in their daily intake. This can be done either by prescribing these separately as medicaments, or by adding them to certain of the feeds during the day.

The requirements for gastrostomy feeding are no different from those of naso-gastric tube feeding; the feed is merely being delivered by another route. Jejunostomy feeding, on the other hand, poses a completely different problem, and is beyond the scope of this book.

E

TABLE III

Example 1 Protein 37 gm.
Calories 1000.

Constituent	Amount gm.	oz.	Protein gm.	Fat gm.	Carbohydrate gm.
Complan (Glaxo)	90	3	27·9	14·4	39·6
Evaporated Milk	120	4	9·4	10·1	14·8
Fat Emulsion	30	1	—	15·0	—
Glucose	75	2½	—	—	68·3
Water to	1000				
			37·3	39·5	122·7

Add daily Vitamins and Iron = Vitamin B Complex—2 mg. Aneurine
2 mg. Riboflavine
10 mg. Nicotinic
Acid

Ascorbic Acid   200 mg.
Ferrous Fumarate   100 mg. t.i.d.
Vitamin A   2500 units
Vitamin D   500 units

Five feeds of 200 ml.

Example 2 Protein 56 gm.
Calories 1500.

Constituent	Amount gm.	oz.	Protein gm.	Fat gm.	Carbohydrate gm.
Complan (Glaxo)	150	5	46·5	24·0	66·0
Evaporated Milk	120	4	9·4	10·1	14·8
Fat Emulsion	45	1½	—	22·5	—
Glucose	120	4	—	—	109·2
Water to	1500				
			55·9	56·6	190·0

Add daily Vitamins and Iron as in Example 1.

Five feeds of 300 ml.

Example 3 Protein 74 gm.
        Calories 2000.

Constituent	Amount gm.	Amount oz.	Protein gm.	Fat gm.	Carbohydrate gm.
Complan (Glaxo)	180	6	55·8	28·8	79·2
Evaporated Milk	240	8	18·7	20·2	29·5
Fat Emulsion	60	2	—	30·0	—
Glucose	150		—	—	136·5
Water to	2000				
			74·5	79·0	245·2

Add daily Vitamins and Iron = Vitamin B Complex—4 mg. Aneurine
                                                  4 mg. Riboflavine
                                                  20 mg. Nicotinic
                                                                Acid
                    Ascorbic Acid   400 mg.
                    Ferrous Fumarate   200 mg. t.i.d.
                    Vitamin D   500 units
                    Vitamin A   2500 units

Five feeds of 400 ml.

Caloric Value of constituents used per 100 grammes:

Constituents	Protein	Fat	Carbohydrate
Complan	31·0	16·0	44·0
Evaporated Milk, e.g. Carnation	7·8	8·4	12·3
Fat Emulsion	—	50·0	—
Glucose	—	—	91·0

Example 3 *continued overleaf*

Example: It is desired to give a protein intake of 74 grammes and a calorie intake of 2000.

Constituent	Amount	Protein	Fat	Carbo-hydrate
	gm.	gm.	gm.	gm.

1. Calculate the protein

Complan	180	55·8	28·8	79·2
Evaporated Milk	240	18·7	20·2	29·5
		74·5	49·0	108·7

2. Calculate 35 per cent total calories.
$$\frac{35 \times 2000}{100} = 710$$

3. Calculate the fat provided by the protein foods.
49 grammes fat =
49 × 9 = 441 cals.

4. Fat to be supplied =
710 − 441 = 269
No. gm. fat =
$$\frac{269}{9} = 29·6(30)$$

Fat Emulsion	60		30·0	
			79·0	

5. Calculate the caloric value of the constituents so far provided.
74·5 × 4 + 79·0 × 9 + 108·7 × 4 = 1444

6. Add additional pure carbohydrate to provide the remainder of the calories.
2000 − 1444 = 556
Each gramme of carbohydrate gives 4 calories; therefore, 556 calories provided by
$$\frac{556 \text{ gm.}}{4} = 139 \text{ gm.}$$
Carbohydrate

Glucose	150			136·5
				245·2

Therefore, the total calories provided (taken to the nearest whole number) =

Protein	=	75 × 4 =	300 Cals.
Fat	=	79 × 9 =	711 Cals.
Carbohydrate	=	245 × 4 =	980 Cals.
			1991 Cals.

BIBLIOGRAPHY

Arney, G. K., Pearson, E. & Sutherland, A. B. (1960). *Ann. Surg.* **152**, 77.
Beck, M. E. (1965). *Nutrition and Dietetics for Nurses*, 2nd ed. Edinburgh: Livingstone.
Blake, E. G. & Wright, H. F. (1963). *Essentials of Paediatric Nursing*. London: Pitman.
Bromley, D. & Burston, W. R. (1966). The Pierre-Robin syndrome. *Nurs. Times*, **62**, 1717.
Dennison, W. M. (1968). *Surgery in Infancy and Childhood*, 2nd ed. Edinburgh: Livingstone.
Moyer, C. A. (1955). *Surgery*, **38**, 806.
Taverner, D. (1961). *Physiology for Nurses*, chaps. 4 & 5. London: English Universities Press.

CHAPTER VIII

ADMINISTRATION OF MEDICINES

The Pharmacy and Poisons Act; the Dangerous Drugs Act; rules for the administration of medicines; oral administration; rectal administration; hypodermic injection; intramuscular injection; inhalations; weights and measures.

THE DANGEROUS DRUGS ACT, PHARMACY AND POISONS ACT, AND RULES FOR THE ADMINISTRATION OF MEDICINES

WHEN administering drugs, the nurse must be fully aware of her responsibility. Laws have been made to protect both the nurse and the patient. These laws regulate the supply, storage and administration of the various drugs. Most hospitals have their own specific rules concerning the labelling, use, and storage of drugs regulated by the Dangerous Drugs Act, the Poisons Act and Therapeutic Substances Act. Additons are made to the list of drugs affected by these Acts from time to time. The Statutes concerned are:

The Pharmacy and Poisons Act 1933 and subsequent orders and regulations of 1949; 1960.

This Act provides for the registration of sellers of poisons, the distribution, sale and use of certain poisons. The Poisons List was drawn up in a number of schedules of which the first and fourth schedules are of interest to nurses.

Schedule I includes a large number of drugs such as arsenic, atropine, curare, strychnine, mercaptopurine, opium. These drugs must be kept in a locked cupboard and the amount checked before administration. To be able to purchase these substances, the chemist must know the purchaser who is required to sign the poison register.

Schedule IV includes many drugs used in medical and veterinary science. These substances may only be supplied on the prescription of a registered medical or veterinary practitioner. The prescription also has to state whether and how often it may be repeated. The drugs in this schedule include barbiturates, carbromal meprobamate, thyroid gland. As new drugs are discovered, these are added from time to time. All drugs included in the poisons list must be clearly and correctly labelled. Drugs for internal administration should be kept in a separate cupboard from those used for external application.

The Dangerous Drugs Act 1920 and subsequent orders and regulations.

This Act aims to control the sale and use of narcotic drugs of addiction. These include opium and its derivatives, Indian hemp (cannabis), cocaine, morphine, heroin, pethidine, etc. Regulations laid down in the Dangerous Drugs Act regarding the prescribing, storage and use of Dangerous Drugs in hospitals must be adhered to. Some of these include:

1. The drugs can only be obtained on a prescription signed by a registered medical practitioner.
2. The drug can only be given to the patient for whom it has been prescribed.
3. The details of the drug and doses administered to each patient must be written in ink in a special Dangerous Drugs Book.
4. All dangerous drugs must be kept in a separate locked cupboard and the key kept on the person of the sister or her deputy.
5. Regular inspection of the Dangerous Drugs cupboard must be made by the pharmacist.
6. The Dangerous Drugs Book must be kept for two years.

Further recommendations have been made by the Joint Sub-Committee on the Control of Dangerous Drugs and Poisons in Hospital. These include the following:

1. Drugs should not be administered without a written prescription except in a real emergency, and in such cases the administration should be recorded on the treatment sheet by the nurse, and confirmed by a doctor within twenty-four hours.
2. It is also recommended that every medicine, whether or not it be a Dangerous Drug or Schedule I poison, should be checked by a second person against the prescription at the bedside immediately before administration.

Therapeutic Substances Act

These include antibiotics and therapeutic substances such as heparin, corticotrophin and vaccines. These are only available on prescriptions signed by a registered medical practitioner.

GUIDING RULES FOR THE ADMINISTRATION OF MEDICINES

When giving medicines, the following rules and recommendations will help to prevent errors and their consequences.

1. The nurse who is administering medicines must not be interrupted or attend to other matters. The greatest care and concentration is required.
2. The prescription is read carefully, and the nurse checks that it is the correct patient. The medicine ordered, the dose and times it is to be given, should be written clearly on the patient's own prescription chart. It is important to ascertain that the medicine has not already been given.
3. When there is any doubt about a drug it must not be given until somebody in authority has been consulted.
4. It has been recommended (Joint Sub-Committee on the Control of Dangerous Drugs and Poisons in Hospitals 1958) that every medicine should be checked against the prescription chart at the bedside immediately before administration. This means that two persons should participate in the medicine round though this may not always be possible.
5. Where possible, the medicine must be examined to make sure that no deterioration has taken place. It is important to read any literature accompanying the drug so as to ascertain the mode of administration; e.g., some medicines should not be given with an acid substance. It will also indicate the method of storing the drug and its stability; e.g., streptomycin should be used within one week if kept at room temperature or one month if kept at temperature below 4°C or 39·2°F. The date of dispensing medicine must be recorded on the bottle and checked to ensure if it is still stable before administering it.
6. When giving drugs like digitalis, it is important to check the apex beat of the patient before and after the drug has been given. This is done because the toxic effect of the drug may

lead to undue slowing of the heart rate. This will indicate that the drug may have to be omitted. If allergic symptoms, such as urticaria, have occurred, the fact must be reported before the causative drug is repeated.

7. The required dose is poured out or prepared. The medicine is given, and recorded on the recording sheet.

8. When pouring medicines from the bottle, the labelled side is held uppermost and the bottle is cleaned immediately after use. Should the label become soiled, the bottle or container should be returned to the pharmacy.

9. Medicine cupboards should be checked daily and only those medicines kept which are required for the patients present in the ward. Any medicines not required should be returned to the pharmacy.

ADMINISTRATION OF MEDICINE

Drugs may be absorbed by different routes

The route used depends on the condition of the child, the speed of action required, and the nature of the drug. It is decided by the doctor. Nurses may give medicines by the following routes:

1. Oral administration.
2. Rectal administration.
3. Inhalation.
4. Hypodermic injection.
5. Intramuscular injection.

Principles involved

1. Patience to find the simplest and most pleasant way of giving medicine to the child.

2. Accuracy to ensure that the correct amount of the ordered preparation is given to the correct patient at the correct time.

3. Knowledge of the action and the reaction of drugs, and the danger of sensitivity to the person giving the drug.

4. Understanding of the methods of absorption.

5. The ability to calculate doses and knowledge of tables before medicines can be given.

ORAL ADMINISTRATION

Oral preparations may be in the form of solutions, mixtures, emulsions, powders, granules, tablets, capsules or cachets.

REASON. It is the simplest and most convenient method, providing the child can swallow and the action of the drug is not diminished or destroyed by gastric juices.

PREPARATION OF THE CHILD. Older children usually show a great pride in their ability to take their medicine, but it is always necessary to find the simplest and the most pleasant way. Special paediatric preparations are available which are more palatable and should not present difficulties. If unpleasantly flavoured medicine has to be given, it can be disguised, or tablets which cannot be swallowed whole can be crushed and mixed with something pleasant such as rose hip syrup. It is essential that the nurse remains with the child until the drug has been swallowed. Not all children will swallow something just to make them better and if given the chance are quite liable to hide tablets under the pillow, or even give them to someone else. Praise for medicine well taken is very important.

BABIES. The nurse washes and dries her hands, and where necessary puts on the gown and whenever possible lifts the infant out of the cot. The infant should be held firmly with the outer arm of the baby restrained and the inner arm tucked well out of the way. The infant is allowed to suck the medicine from a spoon or from a special dropper. It must not be forced into the baby's mouth as it will lead to spluttering and spitting. If a large quantity of medicine has to be given, one quarter of a teaspoonful is given at a time, and the spoon held in readiness to collect any medicine which might be ejected; it is then given again. Water given afterwards helps to rinse the baby's mouth, removes the strange taste, and ensures that the drug has been swallowed.

TODDLERS. A careful approach is essential. If possible, the child should be sitting up, the nurse playing and talking with him first while she ties on the bib. This is time well spent and the child is thus prepared. If these preliminaries are not carried out, such as the child being wakened suddenly and the medicine given immediately, he may reject it or spit it out.

The nurse's approach with children of all ages is important. This is especially so the first time a medicine is given. Time taken and patience exercised will be rewarded.

Trolley for Administration of Oral Medicine

REQUIREMENTS:

1. Medicine glasses graduated in millilitres.
2. Receptacle with spoons.
3. Bottle with sterile water for babies.
4. Jug with orange juice or milk and tumblers.
5. Sweets.
6. Bowl with hot water for washing medicine glasses.
7. Bowl with cold water for rinsing medicine glasses.
8. Drugs
9. Prescription sheets (if used).
10. Disposable towels.

METHOD. The guiding rules of administering medicines should be followed carefully. The method will vary with the type of drug; i.e. whether in liquid form or as a solid. Some children may not be able to swallow tablets whole; these may be crushed between two spoons, but care should be taken not to lose any part of the tablet in the crushing process. A sweet or drink should be given if this is permissible and care taken to ensure that all the drug has been swallowed. Medicines should not be given at meal times unless specially ordered. It is recommended that medicine is given when the stomach is empty. Should this cause any gastric upset, milk may be given with the drug.

As each new drug comes on the market, literature is provided by the drug firms and it is important that these leaflets are read by the nursing staff. They will give the nurse instructions as to the most effective way the drug can be given. Some drugs, such as Chloromycetin Palmitate, must not be given with any other liquid as a chemical change occurs altering the active principle. Individual drugs and their reactions cannot all be mentioned here, far less remembered by the reader.

Knowledge of drugs, the dose for different age-groups, their action and possibilities of reaction and side effects are important. Much can be learnt from a medicine round and it is essential to learn about new drugs as they come into use.

When the medicine round has been completed, bottles are cleansed and all medicines returned to their respective places.

The amount of drugs left should be noted to ensure an adequate supply for twenty-four hours. Drugs must be kept out of reach of children at all times and trays and trolleys are never left in the ward unattended. The advantage of using a specially designed trolley is that it can be locked. This is of particular importance, when the nurse is required to attend to some emergency during the medicine round, thereby ensuring that children will not touch or take any drugs on the trolley.

AFTER CARE OF THE CHILD. Recognition and reporting of any side effects of medicines is of paramount importance.

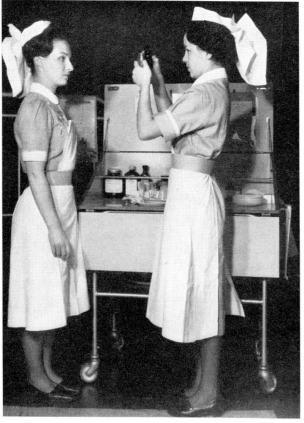

FIG. 23
Administration of medicines. Care and concentration.

RECTAL ADMINISTRATION

REASONS:

1. As an alternative to the oral route in the following circumstances:

    (*a*) To give a drug which would be unpleasant to take orally.

    (*b*) To give a drug to an unconscious or non-cooperative patient.

2. To obtain a local response, as with laxative suppositories.

3. For rectal anaesthetic administration.

PREPARATION AND CARE OF THE CHILD. This is dependent on the type of drug to be administered. If possible, adequate explanation is given. The child should have voided urine and the rectum must be empty of faeces before injecting the drug if anything other than a laxative suppository is to be given.

It is important to remember that if the drug to be given is a basal narcotic anaesthetic, permission must be obtained from the parents and the child prepared as for general anaesthetic. The dose of such drugs is calculated by the body weight, therefore an accurate weight of the child must be obtained.

REQUIREMENTS FOR RECTAL ADMINISTRATION OF A DRUG IN FLUID FORM:

1. Medicine glass with measured and checked amount of drug, standing in a gallipot of warm water.

2. 20 ml. syringe, or funnel and tubing—catheter size 12 F.G. or 6 E.G.

3. Swabs.

4. Lubricant—KY jelly or petroleum jelly.

5. Water-repellent sheet.

6. Receptacle for used equipment.

7. Receptacle for disposable equipment.

METHOD. The drug is checked at the bedside with the chart. If a dangerous drug is being given, the necessary rules of the Dangerous Drugs Act must be observed.

If the nurse is right-handed, it is easier to place the patient comfortably in the left lateral position; if left-handed, vice versa. The bed is protected with the water-repellent sheet and the child kept adequately covered. One nurse should distract the child's attention with a book or toy. The second nurse assembles the apparatus, lightly lubricates the catheter and fills the apparatus with fluid to eject air. The catheter is introduced into the rectum for three to four inches in an upward and slightly forward direction. The funnel should be held just about the level of the buttocks and the fluid allowed to run in very slowly. When all the drug has been given (it may take five minutes to give 30 ml.) the catheter is left in for one minute while the buttocks are compressed. The catheter is gently removed.

AFTER CARE. If the substance given is a basal narcotic, the anaesthetising effect is very rapid. The child must never be left alone and is cared for as any child who has been given a general anaesthetic. Care should be taken to ensure that the substance is retained, except when a local response is desired. The foot of the bed can be elevated when 60 ml. or more of a substance has been given.

INTRODUCTION OF SUPPOSITORY

A suppository consists of gelatinous material which melts when in contact with body heat and releases the drug. Various drugs may be given by this method. The introduction of laxative suppositories has largely taken the place of enemata.

REQUIREMENTS:

1. Lubricant—KY jelly or petroleum jelly.
2. Finger cots or disposable gloves.
3. Suppository.
4. Receptacle for disposable items.
5. Water-repellent sheet, where necessary.

METHOD. Suppositories are painless to introduce and, therefore, should hold no terror for the child. An explanation is given and his co-operation sought. The child is placed comfortably on his side, the suppository is lubricated, and then inserted into the rectum with the protected finger until it is no longer felt.

AFTER CARE. The child should not be left without means of going to the toilet, or obtaining a bedpan quickly when required. The suppository is normally effective about half an hour after insertion. The resultant bowel action should be inspected and reported, and the child's toilet completed.

HYPODERMIC INJECTION
Drugs may be administered by this method:
1. When vomiting is present.
2. Where rapid action is desired.
3. Where the drug may be rendered ineffective by the action of the digestive juices.

PRINCIPLES INVOLVED
1. Knowledge of anatomy of the site; e.g., no blood vessels or nerve endings in the epidermis, but it is rich in lymph derived from the dermis. Nerve endings and blood vessels are present in subcutaneous tissue. The more superficial the injection, the slower the rate of absorption which occurs through the lymphatic system.
2. Reason for inserting the needle at an angle of 25°. This is to ensure that the injection is not given deeper than subcutaneous tissue.
3. Knowledge of aseptic technique.
4. Knowledge of drugs. Certain drugs because of their chemical effect on the tissues must never be given subcutaneously, due to the danger of necrosis of the tissues.
5. Importance of aiding dispersal of the injected fluid by massage.

PREPARATION AND CARE OF THE CHILD. Adequate explanation and truthfulness are essential. Two nurses will be required; one to prepare and comfort the child, expose the appropriate site and hold him still, and the other to give the drug. When the syringe is charged before arrival at the bedside, the development of tension is reduced to a minimum. The child is less likely to be afraid if he cannot see the syringe.

REQUIREMENTS:
Sterile equipment :
1. Small swabs.
2. Container with cleansing lotion or Mediswabs.
3. Disposable syringe (1 or 2 ml.) and needles No. 17.
4. Receptacle for disposable items.

Additional equipment :
5. File.
6. Drug.
7. Prescription sheet.

METHOD. The nurse washes and dries her hands. The needle is then connected to the syringe, keeping the needle point sheathed until the syringe is ready to be charged. Forceps are required if disposable equipment is not used. The rubber top of the bottle is cleaned with a swab soaked in cleansing fluid; alternatively, the vial containing the drug is opened. When a glass vial is opened, care is required to keep the fingers well away from the neck of the vial. A swab may be wrapped round the neck of the vial as a precaution.

When the syringe is charged and all the air excluded, the drug should be checked and taken to the bedside in a covered receptacle

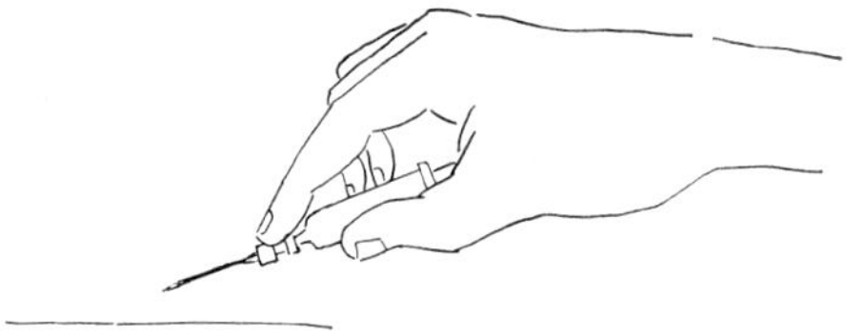

FIG. 24
Hypodermic injection demonstrating the angle
of the needle in relation to the skin.

with a cleansing and a dry swab. At the bedside, the drug is checked again with the chart and it must be confirmed that it is the correct child. As far as possible, the syringe should be kept out of sight. The assistant exposes the upper outer aspect of the arm, or other appropriate site, the skin is cleansed and held taut with one hand, while the syringe is held in the other hand, with the bevel of the needle uppermost. The needle is introduced through the skin at an angle of approximately 25 degrees (Fig. 24). It should penetrate into the subcutaneous tissue for approximately one-quarter inch. The piston is withdrawn slightly to make sure that the needle is not in a blood vessel and the drug is gently injected. The dry swab is then placed over the site of the insertion of the needle and the needle withdrawn. The area is gently massaged in an upward direction to aid the dispersal of the drug. After the procedure, the syringe and needle are disposed of as suggested on page 33. The administration of the drug should then be recorded.

AFTER CARE OF THE CHILD. Most small children will cry either just as the needle is inserted or while the drug is injected. Immediately after the proceedings, he should if possible be picked up and always given some love and comfort. He should never be left to cry himself to sleep. Praise should be given to an older child for co-operation.

INTRAMUSCULAR INJECTION

Drugs are administered by this method for the following reasons:

1. To obtain a rapid action.

2. When the child is unable to take an oral preparation, either because of some physical disability or because the preparation will not be absorbed by the gastro-intestinal tract.

3. When the substance to be given is irritating to the sub-cutaneous tissues.

PRINCIPLES INVOLVED

1. The understanding of the child's natural fear and methods of overcoming this by trust and kindness is the basis of a good technique.

2. Knowledge of anatomy of the sites and the risks involved. The upper outer quadrant of the buttock provides a good muscle and an area where blood vessels and nerves are least likely to be involved (Fig. 25). Alternatively the outer aspect of the thigh can be used.

3. Understanding of the method of absorption of drugs. Muscle tissue is highly vascular and absorption is therefore rapid.

4. Knowledge of aseptic technique.

5. Careless use of antibiotics may produce strains of micro-organisms showing resistance to the antibiotic used. Ejecting antibiotics into the atmosphere is a practice to be avoided. When using rubber sealed single dose bottles, air equivalent in volume to the amount of fluid to be withdrawn is injected into the bottle and the syringe then charged with the drug. It is easier to withdraw the drug by this method, as it avoids a negative pressure in the bottle and lessens the risk of contaminating the atmosphere or hands with antibiotics.

6. Drug Allergies. Allergic dermatitis may be caused by the drug coming repeatedly in contact with a nurse's skin. Gloves should be worn by all who have a predisposition to such a condition and great care must be taken when administering the drug.

7. Danger of anaphylactic reaction. The patient may be allergic to the drug. If given by intramuscular injection, it may cause nausea or vomiting, marked skin rash or other allergic manifestations. Should the drug be given in error into a vein of such a

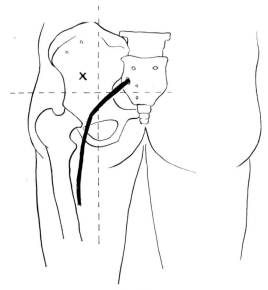

FIG. 25

This demonstrates the anatomical position of the sciatic nerve and the method of determining the point at which an intramusclar injection is safest. The longitudinal line is taken as being from the ischial tuberosity to the iliac crest and the transverse line as midway between the fold of the buttocks below the ischial tuberosity and the upper limit of the iliac crest.

patient, he may collapse and require immediate resuscitation. Adrenalin 1 in 1000 must always be available for such an emergency, and medical aid summoned.

PREPARATION OF THE CHILD. Adequate explanation and absolute truthfulness are essential. It is folly to mislead a child by saying it will not hurt. The child can be reassured that the injection will be much less painful if he lies still and is quite limp and relaxed.

Two nurses will be required, one to prepare and comfort the child, expose the appropriate site and hold him still, the other to administer the drug.

REQUIREMENTS:

Tray contains sterile equipment :
1. Small swabs.
2. Container with cleansing lotion or Mediswab.
3. Disposable syringe of desired size and needles No. 1 or No. 12 for infants.
4. Receptacle for disposable items.

Additional equipment :
5. File.
6. Drug.
7. Ampoule of sterile water (if necessary).
8. Prescription sheet.

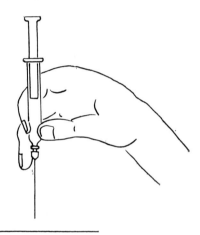

FIG. 26

Intramuscular injection, demonstrating the method of holding the syringe and needle. Note the position of the middle finger to prevent the needle being introduced up to the hilt.

METHOD. The nurse washes and dries her hands, connects the syringe and needle which is kept sheathed. The cap of the bottle containing the drug is then cleansed with a swab soaked in the cleansing fluid. When a single dose is used, air equivalent in volume to the amount of fluid to be withdrawn is injected into the bottle and the syringe is then charged with the drug. Air from the syringe is expelled into the vial. A minute globule should remain to fill the needle on completion of injection. Alternatively, if the drug is in a vial the nurse opens it, keeping her hands well away from the neck of the vial, and charges the syringe. When the syringe is charged, the drug should be checked and taken to the bedside in a covered receptacle containing a cleansing and a dry swab. At the bedside, the drug is checked again with the chart and it must be confirmed that it is the correct child. As far as possible, the syringe should be kept out of sight. The site is cleansed, the skin held taut and pulled downwards. The needle is inserted at right angles to the skin (Fig. 26) as far as 2-3 cm. from the hilt. The piston is withdrawn slightly. If blood appears, the injection should not be given. The needle is withdrawn then reinserted and tested again by withdrawing the piston. The fluid is then injected slowly. A swab is applied over the point of insertion and the needle is withdrawn. Using gentle pressure the area is massaged with the swab to aid dispersal of the drug. After the procedure the syringe and needle are disposed of as suggested on page 33. The administration of the drug should then be recorded.

PRINCIPLES OF TECHNIQUE:

1. The needle is not inserted up to the hilt because of the danger of breaking should the child jerk suddenly. In this eventuality it could not be recovered without operation. This must be remembered when selecting the size of the needle to be used.

2. The needle is inserted quickly as this reduces pain to the minimum.

3. The piston is withdrawn slightly after insertion of the needle to ensure that it has not penetrated a blood vessel.

The dangers of giving drugs intravenously, should an allergy exist, have already been described.

4. The air bubble in the syringe will enter the needle after the injection has been given, thus ensuring that there will be minimal leakage of the drug into the subcutaneous tissues as the needle is withdrawn.

5. The skin and subcutaneous tissue is pulled downwards before the insertion of the needle. When the skin is released, the path taken by the needle is no longer straight and, therefore, leakage of the drug along this channel cannot occur. Leakage would cause considerable discomfort if the drug is irritating to the subcutaneous tissues. An iron preparation could cause staining of the skin.

6. Slow injection of the drug permits dispersal of the fluid with less pain. Massaging the area after injection aids dispersal.

7. A needle 38 mm. long will penetrate muscle if injected for two-thirds of its length. Such a needle has also an adequate bore to enable drugs to be given with less force and thus reduces pain. The use of a smaller needle unless for an infant under one year is dangerous as it is more easily broken and less likely to penetrate the muscle deeply enough for the absorption of the drug. Considerable pain and reaction in the subcutaneous tissue is caused by certain drugs if not given correctly.

8. The recommended amount and type of fluid must be used for dissolving the drug to be given. If less fluid is used, the material injected is more concentrated and, therefore, more irritating to the tissues. It ceases to be an isotonic solution and will cause considerable pain and may lead to tissue necrosis.

An intramuscular injection can be comparatively painless if the technique is good. Several cardinal rules must be observed to acquire a good technique:

1. The child must be relaxed, and held expertly and gently.

2. The needle is quickly inserted and quickly withdrawn though the drug is given slowly by good piston control.

3. After the drug is given, the area must be gently massaged.

4. When a course of injections is given, the sites must be chosen according to a definite rotation.

5. Injections of over 2 ml. in infants and 3 ml. in the older child should be given in divided doses using two sites.

INHALATION

REASON. Inhalation provides relief in certain types of respiratory distress. Aerosol drugs are used which have a local effect on inflamed tissue and may be given in such conditions as bronchitis, laryngitis, laryngeal stridor or asthma.

Inhalation of vapour will moisten and loosen secretions, relieving distress and lessening the danger of respiratory obstruction in laryngo-tracheo-bronchitis, fibrocystic disease of the pancreas and the immediate post-operative period of tracheostomy.

Methods of Inhalation

1. INCUBATOR. The Oxygenaire incubator and the 'Isolette' of Air-Shields, Inc. can provide up to 100 per cent humidity. The

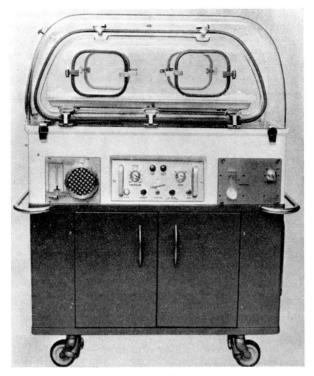

FIG. 27
Oxygenaire incubator. (By kind permission of Vickers Ltd.)

degree of humidity is recorded on a hygrometer and can be altered as necessary. The incubators have a controlled regulating mechanism and infants can, therefore, be nursed without restrictive clothing. The tray the infant is nursed on may be tilted as desired. Oxygen can be given as necessary (Fig. 27).

2. CROUPETTE OR HUMIDAIRE. Types of tent in which the child can be nursed in maximum humidity. Both tents can be used with or without oxygen and achieve 100 per cent humidity at an even cool temperature. The vapour produced is very fine and penetrates the entire respiratory tract (Fig. 28). A nebulising attachment can be used to administer aerosol drugs.

3. CROUPAIRE. A compact, light-weight, portable machine which is a cool vapour humidifier. It is safe for use with children. No tent is required and it will operate without attention for ten

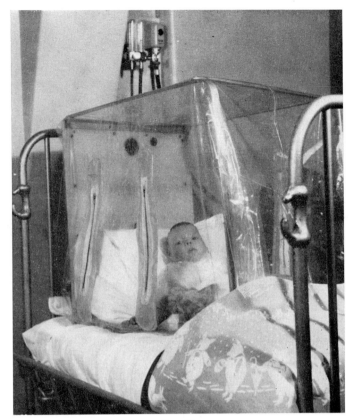

FIG. 28
Croupette

hours. The Croupaire can be placed on a locker top with the vapour directed at the child (Fig. 29).

4. HYDROJETTE. This is a cool vapour humidifier. It is fixed to a small trolley and has an adjustable counterpoised arm which provides adequate vapour without mask or tent. It is safe with children. The Hydrojette can be used with a fitted collar for the use of a child with a tracheostomy tube. The collar has a small window which is easily adjusted when suction is required. The collar causes no discomfort and is not alarming for the child (Fig. 30). (See Tracheostomy, Chapter XII.)

5. STEAM TENT. The use of a steam kettle and tent will give a warm atmosphere of high humidity.

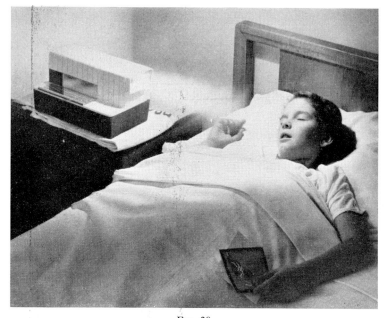

FIG. 29

Croupaire. (By kind permission of the Medical Supply Association Ltd.)

6. NEBULISERS. Used to administer aerosol drugs for their local effect on the nasal passages or the bronchial muscles.

7. INHALER. For the administration of volatile drugs which have a local effect on the respiratory tract.

The Diapump is used with the Croupette and the Hydrojette. The Oxygenaire Air Compressor is used with the Humidaire. These machines produce compressed filtered air which is forced through distilled water to form a fine spray of water vapour. This is more economical than using oxygen which would have to be run at a much higher rate than normal to achieve the necessary pressure.

Some models have a suction apparatus which is essential at the bedside when nursing any child who has a severe respiratory infection.

Adequate maintenance of these machines is essential. Leaflets are provided and instructions should be followed.

One of the possible causes of failure is when the glass jars do not fit correctly. These should be checked and screwed carefully into the sockets. In the Diapump, one jar contains the filter which,

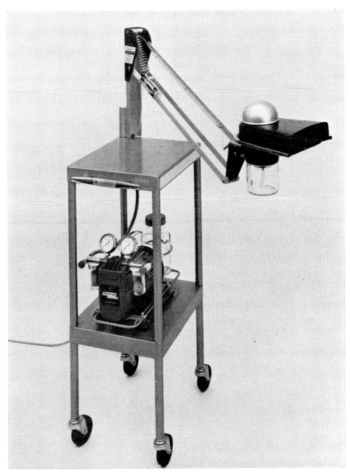

FIG. 30

Hydrojette, showing Diapump with suction. (By kind permission of Air-Shields Inc.)

when the wool is blackened at both ends, is no longer effective. The other contains a cork ball which occludes the entrance to the mechanism should overflow of water occur when suction is used.

Croupette and Humidaire

PREPARATION OF THE CHILD. It is most important that the child should not be alarmed or frightened when the tent is first erected around him. Fear will cause distress, and consequently greater respiratory embarrassment. It is important, therefore, to explain what is happening if he is old enough to understand. Children of all ages should not be left alone until they have settled and care should be taken that they can see those around them. A favourite toy can be put inside the croupette provided that it is not a mechanical sparking toy, particularly if oxygen is to be used (Dangers in the use of oxygen, Chapter XII).

REQUIREMENTS:

1. Croupette or Humidaire.
2. Diapump or Air Compressor.
3. Distilled water.
4. Ice or iced water.
5. Wall thermometer.

METHOD. The tent is erected over the child. The Croupette is ideal for infants though it can be used over the head and shoulders of an older child. The Humidaire is large enough to envelop a cot. The simple directions on the side of the tent can be easily followed. The wall thermometer is placed at the side of the pillow and the child made comfortable with one or two pillows. To obtain 100 per cent humidity, the side dial should register 10 lb. pressure per square inch. Excellent diagrammatic instruction books are provided with these tents and these should be studied carefully.

IMPORTANT POINTS ON MAINTENANCE:

1. Care must be taken not to occlude the portal of entry of humid air. This may easily occur with the Croupette if pillows are propped up against the back.

2. The ledge on the plastic back of the Croupette is to allow excess moisture to drain out. This gutter should be kept clear. Pillows will become wet quickly if allowed to rest up against it.

3. Adequate ice, or ice-cold water, is necessary in the back chamber to keep the Croupette cool.

AFTER USE. Disinfection is carried out as for an oxygen tent. With the Croupette, the glass jar is emptied, washed and dried, and the component parts in the jar are removed and rinsed under the running tap. A soft brush may be used to cleanse them if necessary.

The filter of the Humidaire is cleaned in the same way. Warmed distilled water is put into the humidifier for a few minutes at maximum flow to dissolve any solid residue that may have accumulated inside the humidifier jet.

The Croupette, Croupaire, Hydrojette and Diapump are manufactured in Great Britain by Air-Shields (U.K.) Inc. and marketed solely by the Medical Supply Association. The Humidaire and Air Compressor are manufactured by Oxygenaire, London.

Children suffering from fibrocystic disease of the pancreas have thick viscid mucus which, without adequate treatment, may occlude the alveoli of the lungs. With expert physiotherapy and nursing care many of these children can be looked after at home, avoiding long periods in hospital. A humid environment is helpful

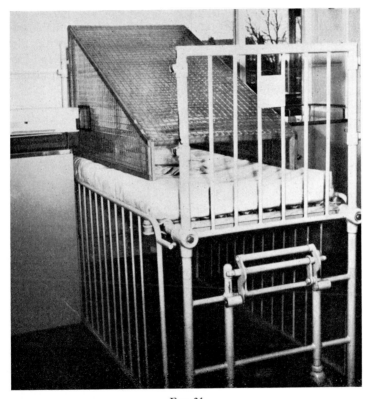

FIG. 31

The Pendlebury Hood for use with Croupaire designed for home use by Miss F. Floyd. (Reprinted by kind permission of The Royal Manchester Children's Hospital.)

prior to physiotherapy to loosen the thick mucous material.
Figure 31 demonstrates a hood which has been designed for home
use with the Croupaire. This has been designed by a ward sister
at the Royal Manchester Hospital, Pendlebury. Claritex 1-in.
light-weight mesh is used covered on both sides with polythene.
Cost of the hood is minimal.

Steam Tent

This method of providing a humid atmosphere has been largely
superseded by the Croupette or Humidaire, but it may still be
used when these are not immediately available.

This tent is made with sheets and screens. Steam from a special
long-spouted kettle is directed from a safe distance into the tent.

PREPARATION OF THE CHILD. The child is placed in the most
comfortable position in bed, usually propped up with three
pillows to facilitate easier breathing. Light bedclothes and loose
fitting clothes should be used and adequate explanation given to
the child to allay fear.

REQUIREMENTS:

1. One or two screens according to size.
2. One or two sheets.
3. Safety pins.
4. Steam kettle (electric).
5. Low table and tray for kettle.
6. If ordered, tincture of benzoin co. and measure. Many
physicians feel that steam is as effective and less unpleasant than
the smell of tincture of benzoin co. which is of doubtful value.
7. Wall thermometer.

METHOD. The tent is erected over the top one-third of the bed.
Sheets should be folded neatly and overhang at least one and a
half feet from the top of the screen at the front. An aperture must
be left at the back of the tent for the spout of the kettle. The
kettle is kept on the table outside the tent and the spout directed
within, well away from the child's face and out of reach of a restless
toddler.

The kettle should be filled with boiling water for quicker effect.
One drachm of tincture of benzoin co. may be added if ordered.

The thermometer is hung inside the tent and the temperature

checked hourly. Excessive warmth will cause further distress to the child through exhaustion. An attempt should be made to maintain a temperature not exceeding 21·1°C or 79°F. The level of water in the kettle is checked at hourly intervals and refilled as necessary.

CARE OF THE CHILD. The child must be protected from scalding at all times. Restraints are necessary for the young or disorientated child. A clear airway must be maintained and the position adopted which will cause the least respiratory embarrassment. Sponging the child and changing of linen should be carried out as necessary.

Nebulisers and Inhalers

The Nelson's inhaler is not recommended for use with children, as it necessitates the use of water at temperatures varying from 71·1°C or 160°F to boiling point.

There are many proprietary nebulisers and inhalers effective in the relief of nasal congestion and for the relief of bronchospasm as in asthma.

Medical orders must be strictly adhered to so far as frequency of use is concerned and it is important to stress, if they are for home use, that other members of the family do not make use of them as they can be a source of infection. The technique of using them should be taught to the child and clearly understood by the parents.

WEIGHTS AND MEASURES

A knowledge of weights and measures is of the utmost importance. Although the imperial system is employed in this country, the metric system is gradually being more widely used. It is important therefore that the nurse should be conversant with both systems and be able to convert from one to the other.

A table of approximate equivalents will also be given which will be of practical value both for domestic use and for the dilution of lotions. Drops vary in size and are a very inaccurate way of measuring volume. Most paediatric medicines have their individual measured droppers and clear instructions are usually issued indicating the amount of drug each drop contains.

IMPERIAL SYSTEM

Weight

Apothecaries:

Pound	Ounces	Drachms	Scruples	Grains
1	12	96	288	5760
	1	8	24	480
		1	3	60
			1	20

Avoirdupois or accurate weight:

Pound	Ounces	Drachms	Grains
1	16	256	7000
	1	16	437·5
		1	27·343

14 pounds = 1 stone.

Volume (fluid)

Gallon	Quarts	Pints	Ounces	Drachms	Minims
1	4	8	160	1280	76800
	1	2	40	320	19200
		1	20	160	9600
			1	8	480
				1	60

METRIC SYSTEM

Weight

1000 microgrammes = 1 milligramme (mg.)
1000 milligrammes = 1 gramme (gm.)
1000 grammes = 1 kilogramme (kg.)

500 grammes $= \frac{1}{2}$ kilogramme = 0·5 kg.
500 milligrammes $= \frac{1}{2}$ gramme = 0·5 gm.
250 milligrammes $= \frac{1}{4}$ gramme = 0·25 gm.
125 milligrammes $= \frac{1}{8}$ gramme = 0·125 gm.
1 milligramme $= \frac{1}{1000}$ gramme = 0·001 gm.

Volume

1000 millilitres = 1 litre
1000 ml. or 1000 cubic centimetres (cc.) = 1 litre
    1 litre of water at 4°C weighs 1 kilogramme
1 cc. of water = 1 ml. and weighs 1 gramme at 4°C

METRIC AND IMPERIAL EQUIVALENTS

1 milligramme =	0·0154	grains
1 gramme	= 15·4	grains
1 ml.	= 16·9	minims
1 litre	= 35·2	fluid ounces

1 grain	= 0·065	grammes
480 grains	= 31·1	grammes
1 minim	= 0·059	millilitres
1 fl. ounce	= 28·4	millilitres

APPROXIMATE IMPERIAL AND METRIC EQUIVALENTS

Volume (fluid)

40 fl. ounces = 1200 ml.	10 fl. ounces =	300 ml.
35 fl. ounces = 1000 ml.	3½ fl. ounces =	100 ml.
20 fl. ounces = 600 ml.	1 fl. ounce =	30 ml.
17 fl. ounces = 500 ml.	½ fl. ounce =	15 ml.

2½ fl. drachms = 10 ml.	10 minims = 0·6 ml.
1 fl. drachm = 4 ml.	8 minims = 0·5 ml.
45 minims = 3·0 ml.	5 minims = 0·3 ml.
30 minims = 2·0 ml.	4 minims = 0·25 ml.
15 minims = 1·0 ml.	3 minims = 0·2 ml.
12 minims = 0·75 ml.	1½ minims = 0·1 ml.

Weight

1 oz. = 30 gm.	10 grains = 600 mg.
½ oz. = 15 gm.	7½ grains = 450 mg.
120 grains = 8 gm.	5 grains = 300 mg.
60 grains = 4 gm.	4 grains = 250 mg.
30 grains = 2 gm.	3 grains = 200 mg.
15 grains = 1 gm.	2½ grains = 150 mg.

$1\frac{1}{2}$ grains	= 100 mg.	$\frac{1}{10}$	grain =	6 mg.
1 grain	= 60 mg.	$\frac{1}{20}$	grain =	3 mg.
$\frac{3}{4}$ grain	= 50 mg.	$\frac{1}{60}$	grain =	1 mg.
$\frac{1}{2}$ grain	= 30 mg.	$\frac{1}{100}$	grain =	0·6 mg.
$\frac{1}{3}$ grain	= 20 mg.	$\frac{1}{120}$	grain =	0·5 mg.
$\frac{1}{4}$ grain	= 15 mg.	$\frac{1}{200}$	grain =	0·3 mg.
$\frac{1}{6}$ grain	= 10 mg.	$\frac{1}{300}$	grain =	0·2 mg.
$\frac{1}{8}$ grain	= 7·5 mg.	$\frac{1}{600}$	grain =	0·1 mg.

COMPARATIVE WEIGHT AND HEIGHT SCALES

When children are admitted to hospital they are weighed and their height is measured. This is part of the physical examination and is an indication of the progress of the individual child.

While in hospital, the frequency of weighing varies with the age and the condition of the child.

Infants up to 1 year old are usually weighed daily. Children from 1 year upwards are usually weighed once a week except in special circumstances; e.g., a child suffering from nephrosis would be weighed more frequently, such as daily or every second day.

Except in special circumstances, children are only measured on admission to hospital.

The weight and height scales may be expressed in either British units or metric units. The Metric system is now gradually superseding the British system. Measurements can readily be converted from one system to the other and conversion tables from the British to the metric system are appended.

WEIGHT

2·2 lb. = 1 kg.
1 oz. = 30 grammes.

Example: Infant's weight is $3\frac{1}{2}$ lb.
and 2·2 lb. = 1 kg.

$$\therefore 3·5 \text{ lb.} = \frac{3·5 \times 1}{2·2}$$

$$= \frac{35}{22} = 1·59 \text{ kg.}$$

WEIGHT CONVERSION TABLE

1·1 lb.	=	½ kg. or 0·5 kg. or 500 grammes			
2·2 lb.	=	1 kg. or 1000 grammes			
3 lb.	=	1·36 kg.	14 lb.	=	6·35 kg.
3½ lb.	=	1·59 kg.	15 lb.	=	6·81 kg.
4 lb.	=	1·81 kg.	16 lb.	=	7·18 kg.
4½ lb.	=	2·04 kg.	17 lb.	=	7·71 kg.
5 lb.	=	2·27 kg.	18 lb.	=	8·18 kg.
5½ lb.	=	2·5 kg.	19 lb.	=	8·63 kg.
6 lb.	=	2·72 kg.	20 lb.	=	9·09 kg.
6½ lb.	=	2·95 kg.	21 lb.	=	9·54 kg.
7 lb.	=	3·18 kg.	22 lb.	–	10·00 kg.
7½ lb.	=	3·40 kg.	23 lb.	=	10·45 kg.
8 lb.	=	3·63 kg.	24 lb.	=	10·90 kg.
8½ lb.	=	3·86 kg.	25 lb.	=	11·66 kg.
9 lb.	=	4·09 kg.	30 lb.	=	13·63 kg.
10 lb.	=	4·5 kg.	35 lb.	=	15·90 kg.
11 lb.	=	5·0 kg.	40 lb.	=	18·18 kg.
12 lb.	=	5·75 kg.	45 lb.	=	20·45 kg.
13 lb.	=	5·9 kg.	50 lb.	=	22·72 kg.

HEIGHT CONVERSION TABLE

1 inch = 2·54 cm.

100 cm. = 1 metre.

Example : Child measures 32 inches

and 1 inch = 2·54 cm.

∴ 32 in. = 32 × 2·54 cm.

= 81·2 cm.

18 in. = 45·72 cm.	30 in. = 76·20 cm.
19 in. = 48·26 cm.	31 in. = 78·74 cm.
20 in. = 50·80 cm.	32 in. = 81·28 cm.
21 in. = 53·34 cm.	33 in. = 83·82 cm.
22 in. = 55·88 cm.	34 in. = 86·36 cm.
23 in. = 58·42 cm.	35 in. = 88·90 cm.
24 in. = 60·96 cm.	36 in. = 91·44 cm.
25 in. = 63·54 cm.	37 in. = 93·98 cm.
26 in. = 66·04 cm.	38 in. = 96·52 cm.
27 in. = 68·58 cm.	39 in. = 99·06 cm.
28 in. = 71·12 cm.	40 in. = 101·60 cm. or 1 metre 1·6 cm.
29 in. = 73·66 cm.	42 in. = 106·68 cm.

F

44 in. = 111·76 cm.	54 in. = 137·16 cm.
46 in. = 116·84 cm.	56 in. = 142·24 cm.
48 in. = 121·92 cm.	58 in. = 147·32 cm.
50 in. = 127·00 cm.	60 in. = 152·40 cm.
52 in. = 132·08 cm.	

DILUTIONS OF LOTIONS

Formula:

Divide the figure representing the weak solution by that representing the stronger solution.

Multiply the amount of weak solution required by the result and the answer is the amount of strong solution to be used.

Example:

Prepare 1 pint carbolic lotion 1 in 80 from stock solution of carbolic lotion 1 in 20.

$$\frac{\text{weak solution 1 in 80}}{\text{strong solution 1 in 20}} = \frac{1}{80} \div \frac{1}{20} = \frac{1}{80} \times \frac{20}{1} = \frac{1}{4}$$

Amount required is 20 ounces $\therefore 20 \times \frac{1}{4} = 5$ ounces.

Take 5 ounces of 1 in 20 carbolic lotion and add 15 ounces of water.

= 20 ounces of 1 in 80 solution.

PERCENTAGE DILUTION OF LOTIONS

Per cent or % (Latin, per centum) means 'for every hundred'.
$\therefore$ 10% meaning 10 out of every 100, is the same thing as

$$\frac{10}{100} \text{ or } \frac{1}{10} \text{ or } 0·1$$

10%	=	100 ml. in 1000 ml. or 1 litre
2½%	=	25 ml. in 1000 ml. or 1 litre
1%	=	10 ml. in 1000 ml. or 1 litre
0·1%	=	1 ml. in 1000 ml. or 1 litre

⅝%	=	1 drachm in 1 pint or 1 in 160
1%	=	96 minims in 1 pint or 1 in 100
2½%	=	½ ounce in 1 pint or 1 in 40
5%	=	1 ounce in 1 pint or 1 in 20
10%	=	2 ounces in 1 pint or 1 in 10

To Make 1% Solution of a Solid the Following Methods are Available:

1. Weigh 1 gramme and make up to 100 ml. with the solvent.
2. Weigh 1 ounce (437·5 gr.) and make up to 100 fl. ounces with the solvent.
3. Weigh 1 grain and make up to 110 minims with the solvent.

To Give Part of a Tablet:

Formula:

$$\frac{\text{What we want}}{\text{What we have}} = \text{Fraction of tablet to be given.}$$

Dissolve the tablet in a number of minims of water, and give the fraction calculated.

Example:

Give $\frac{1}{10}$ grain of morphine from tablet $\frac{1}{6}$ grain.

$$\frac{\text{What we want } \frac{1}{10}}{\text{What we have } \frac{1}{6}} = \frac{1}{10} \div \frac{1}{6} = \frac{1}{10} \times \frac{6}{1} = \frac{3}{5} \text{ of tablet to be given.}$$

Dissolve the tablet grain $\frac{1}{6}$ in 10 minims of water:

$$\therefore \frac{3}{5} \times 10 = 6 \text{ minims of grain } \frac{1}{10} \text{ dose.}$$

Normal saline solution   80 grains of salt in 1 pint of water.
Physiological saline $= 0.9\%$ approx. 1 drachm of salt in 1 pint of water.

COMPARATIVE TEMPERATURE SCALES

Temperature may be measured in either Fahrenheit or Centigrade scale, and it is useful to be able to convert from one scale to the other. Greater use is now being made of the Centigrade scale.

The basic temperatures on both scales are:

(*a*) the melting point of ice or freezing point of water: 0°C and 32°F.
(*b*) the boiling point of water: 100°C and 212°F.

Now since the difference in temperature between the melting point of ice and the boiling point of water is always the same, the number of Centigrade degrees in this range can be equated to the number of Fahrenheit degrees in the same range.

Thus $100°C - 0°C$ is equal to $212°F - 32°F$

i.e. 100 Centigrade degrees $=$ 180 Fahrenheit degrees

or

1 Centigrade degree $=$ 9/5 Fahrenheit degree

and also

1 Fahrenheit degree $=$ 5/9 Centigrade degree

For example:

    $95°F = (95 - 32)$ °F above freezing point on the Fahrenheit scale,

    i.e. $63°F$ above freezing point and $1°F = 5/9°C$

$$\therefore 95°F = \frac{63 \times 5°C}{9} = 35°C$$

From this we get the rule:

To convert Fahrenheit to Centigrade $=$ Subtract 32, multiply by 5 and divide by 9.

To convert Centigrade to Fahrenheit $=$ Multiply by 9, divide by 5 and add 32.

For example:

$$60°C = \frac{60 \times 9}{5} = 108 + 32 = 140°F$$

TEMPERATURE CONVERSION TABLES

° Fahrenheit				° Centigrade	° Centigrade				° Fahrenheit
80	.	.	.	. 26·7	26	.	.	.	. 78·8
81	.	.	.	. 27·2	27	.	.	.	. 80·6
82	.	.	.	. 27·8	28	.	.	.	. 82.4
83	.	.	.	. 28·3	29	.	.	.	. 84·2
84	.	.	.	. 28·9	30	.	.	.	. 86·0
85	.	.	.	. 29·4	31	.	.	.	. 87·8
86	.	.	.	. 30·0	32	.	.	.	. 89·6
87	.	.	.	. 30·6	33	.	.	.	. 91·4
88	.	.	.	. 31·1	34	.	.	.	. 93·2
89	.	.	.	. 31·7	35	.	.	.	. 95·0
90	.	.	.	. 32·2	36	.	.	.	. 96·8
91	.	.	.	. 32·8	37	.	.	.	. 98·6
92	.	.	.	. 33·3	38	.	.	.	. 100·4
93	.	.	.	. 33·9	39	.	.	.	. 102·2
94	.	.	.	. 34·4	40	.	.	.	. 104·0

° Fahrenheit	° Centigrade	° Centigrade	° Fahrenheit
95	35·0	41	105·8
96	35·6	42	107·6
97	36·1	43	109·4
98	36·7	44	111·2
99	37·2	45	113·0
100	37·8	46	114·8
101	38·3	47	116·6
102	38·9	48	118·4
103	39·4	49	120·2
104	40·0	50	122·0
105	40·6		
106	41·1		
107	41·7		
108	42·2		
109	42·8		
110	43·3		
111	43·9		
112	44·4		
113	45·0		
114	45·6		
115	46·1		
116	46·7		
117	47·2		
118	47·8		
119	48·3		
120	48·9		

BIBLIOGRAPHY

Bendall, E. R. D. & Raybould, E. (1965). Basic Nursing, 2nd ed. London: Lewis.

Crooks, J., Clark, C. J., Caie, H. B. & Mason, W. B. (1965). Lancet, 1, 373.

Ellison Nash, D. F. (1965). Principles and Practice of Surgical Nursing, 3rd ed. London: Arnold.

Harmer, B. & Henderson, V. (1955). Principles and Practice of Nursing, 5th ed., chap. 25 & 26. New York: Macmillan.

Hector, W. (1968). Modern Nursing Theory and Practice, chap. 8. London: Heinemann.

Hodgson, R. W. (1962). Every student's guide to the metric system. Nurs. Mirror, 114, 2977.

Ministry of Health (1957). Therapeutic Substances. London: Her Majesty's Stationery Office.

Ministry of Health (1958). Control of Dangerous Drugs and Poisons in Hospital. Central Health Services Council. London: H.M.S.O.

Ministry of Health (1960). The Poison Rules. London: H.M.S.O.

Sykes, M. K. (1962). Oxygen therapy. Nurs. Times, 58, 301.

CHAPTER IX

PROCEDURES RELATING TO THE NERVOUS SYSTEM

Lumbar puncture; cisternal puncture; subdural and ventricular puncture; neurological examination; electroencephalography.

LUMBAR PUNCTURE

REASONS:

This procedure is carried out for the following purposes:
1. Diagnostic: Where infection of the meninges is suspected.
2. To remove cerebro-spinal fluid in an effort to decrease intra-cranial pressure; e.g., hydrocephalus and meningitis.
3. To administer a drug; e.g. penicillin.
4. To administer spinal anaesthesia.
5. For X-ray examination of the ventricles.

PRINCIPLES INVOLVED. The spinal cord ends at the level of the first lumbar vertebra but the meninges, i.e. dura mater, arachnoid and pia mater, are prolonged below it. The subarachnoid space contains cerebro-spinal fluid. A needle is inserted into the space between the third and fourth lumbar vertebrae, where there will be no danger of damage to the spinal cord.

Normal spinal fluid is a clear, colourless fluid, containing not more than five lymphocytes per cm., protein 20-30 mg. per 100 ml., and sugar 50-80 mg. per 100 ml. The total volume is 20 ml., in a newborn infant, increasing with age until it reaches the total of 100-150 ml. in adulthood. The initial pressure is 70-200 mm. of water.

In disease, the amount and type of fluid may be altered and may show the following:

(a) *Clear fluid, but a positive Pandy's test.* Pandy's test is a qualitative test which indicates increase in protein. Spinal fluid protein is increased in most diseases of the central nervous system especially meningitis and subarachnoid haemorrhage.

(b) *Purulent fluid* indicates infection by organisms such as meningococcus, bacillus coli, etc.

(c) Blood may be found in subarachnoid haemorrhage.

The pressure may be raised in hydrocephalus, tumour of the brain or where infection of the meninges is present. This can be accurately recorded only in the older child.

REQUIREMENTS:

Disposable sterile equipment where applicable.
1. Swabs.
2. Cleansing lotions in current use or Mediswabs.
3. 2 prs. dressing forceps.
4. 3 lumbar puncture needles with well-fitting stilettes.
5. Glass manometer and a small piece of rubber tubing (for measuring cerebro-spinal fluid pressure).
6. 2 ml. syringe and hypodermic needles for local anaesthesia; 5 and 10 ml. syringes.
7. Sterile metal stand with sterile test tubes and centrifuge tubes, or specimen bottles.

Additional equipment:

8. Local anaesthesia.
9. Antibiotic or substance to be injected.
10. Phenol 1-15 (for Pandy's test).
11. Receptacle for disposable equipment.
12. Labels.

PREPARATION OF THE CHILD. Sedation may be given to children prior to the procedure. A local anaesthesia may also be given. The child must be prevented from moving during the procedure and this may be achieved by placing the child on his side, the back level with the table edge (Fig. 32). The nurse's right arm is placed under the child's knees, grasping the child's arms. The left arm is placed round his neck bending his back. This increases the intervertebral space, but care must be taken not to flex the head excessively as it might lead to respiratory and circulatory embarrassment. Alternatively, the child may be placed in the sitting position, supported by a nurse.

AFTER CARE. After this procedure, pressure is applied to the puncture site or an adhesive dressing may be applied. Nobecutane is sprayed on to the site; it is sterile and is therefore preferred to collodion. The child is dressed and placed in a warmed bed with one pillow. If headache and vomiting are present, the foot of the bed can be raised and glucose fluids given. If there is any pain in the neck, legs or back, it must be reported; it may be due to bleeding into the theca or to infection.

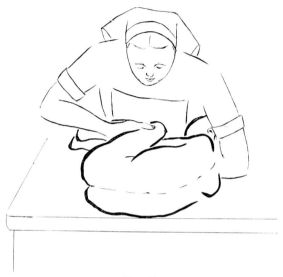

FIG. 32
Position of child for lumbar puncture

CISTERNAL PUNCTURE:

In this procedure a needle is inserted into the cisterna magna. This is the largest of the subarachnoid cisternae or spaces. It lies in the angle between the cerebellum and the medulla and can be reached by passing a needle between the first cervical vertebra and the skull.

This procedure is more dangerous than the lumbar puncture and injury to the medulla may occur, therefore cisternal puncture is seldom used for routine examination of the cerebro-spinal fluid, but where there is a block; i.e., some obstruction in the spinal canal, cisternal puncture is the method of choice. It is done for the same purposes as lumbar puncture and the requirements are the same. Special cisternal puncture needles may be used for the older child.

PREPARATION OF THE CHILD. Pre-operative procedure is the same as for lumbar puncture, but the position of the child is different. The child either lies on his side, the shoulders in vertical line and the head slightly flexed, or he may be in the sitting position with the head slightly flexed. It may be necessary to shave the nape of the neck. During the procedure the child must be held firmly so that no movement takes place. The after care is the same as for lumbar puncture.

Sub-Dural Puncture and Ventricular Puncture

This procedure is carried out to determine the presence of sub-dural haematoma and the presence of a hydrocephalus. If a haematoma is present, the cerebro-spinal fluid will be grossly xanthochromic or bloodstained and will be more abundant. These procedures can only be carried out in infants where the sutures of the skull have not closed. When the sutures and the anterior fontanelle have closed, the procedure is more extensive, requiring burr holes, and is carried out by a neuro-surgeon.

REQUIREMENTS. As for lumbar puncture. A shorter and graduated needle may be used.

PREPARATION OF THE CHILD. The scalp has to be shaved and the child restrained, lying on his back with the top of his head level with the edge of the table. The nurse holds the head, tilting it slightly forward. The needle is inserted into the extreme lateral corner of the anterior fontanelle. When fluid had been withdrawn, firm digital pressure is applied over the punctured areas and the child's head is raised. Pressure must be maintained until no further leakage of cerebro-spinal fluid occurs.

Neurological Examination

The examination aims at testing the efficiency of the nervous system, sensory, motor and reflex. In certain conditions, such as diseases of the nervous system; e.g., hemiplegia, poliomyelitis and new growths either within the spinal cord or brain, the peripheral nerves will be affected.

REQUIREMENTS:

1. Eye drop bottle containing a mydriatic to dilate the pupils.
2. Ophthalmoscope for the examination of the eyes.
3. Tuning fork, to test the sense of hearing.
4. Pin cushion with pins, to test pressure and pain sensations.

5. Patellar hammer, to test the reflexes.
6. Soft brush or a wisp of cotton wool, to test corneal pressure and reflexes.
7. Test tubes containing hot and cold water, to test receptors for heat and cold.
8. Small bottles containing sugar, salt, lemon juice, peppermint, to test the sense of taste.
9. Tape measure. This is used (a) to measure circumference of head where a hydrocephalus is suspected.
    (b) to measure limbs where shortening of one or more limbs is suspected.
10. Skin pencil.
11. Gallipot with cotton wool balls.
12. Receptacle for soiled cotton wool balls.

PREPARATION OF THE CHILD. Co-operation is essential, therefore older children should have the examination explained to them and younger children should be reassured and calmed. Their attention should be taken up with other occupations, such as toys. The child is undressed and covered with a light blanket. For examination of the eyes, dilation may be necessary and the room darkened. Quietness of the surroundings is essential when the sense of hearing is to be tested.

ELECTROENCEPHALOGRAPHY

This is a method of recording the electrical activity of the cortex of the brain. It is an aid to diagnosis in cases where there is a history of recurrent convulsions. It may be of value in the diagnosis of epilepsy and intracranial disease and in defining the area affected by a pathological process.

Electrodes are placed at various positions on the scalp and connected through a valve amplifier to an ink-writing oscillograph. It is carried out in a quiet room. The child should be reassured and, if old enough to understand, it should be explained that this is not a painful procedure. He should be kept as calm and relaxed as possible. Sedation is not desirable as it alters the pattern of the recording, but if it is unavoidable the fact must be recorded.

BIBLIOGRAPHY

Fairburn, B. (1967). Neurosurgery today. *Nurs. Times*, **63**, 3.

Garb, S. & Sporne, P. (1962). *Nurse's Manual of Laboratory Tests*. London: Heinemann.

Ross, J. S. & Wilson, K. J. W. (1968). *Foundations of Anatomy and Physiology*, 3rd ed. Edinburgh: Livingstone.

CHAPTER X

EXAMINATION AND TREATMENT OF EYES

Examination of eyes; application of ointment; application of heat; instillation of eye drops and irrigation of eyes, eye pads.

WHILE a child is in hospital because of some illness or accident, it may be necessary to carry out examination and treatment of his eyes. It is not proposed to deal here with the specialised procedures of an Eye Department, but the frequent attention the child's eyes require while in a general ward justifies a few words on the subject. For example, corneal ulceration may occur in an unconscious or anaesthetised child whose eyes have been left open. This condition may be prevented by ensuring that the eyelids of the child are kept closed and are treated by lubricating the eyes twice daily with an abundance of bland antiseptic ointment.

On the admission of a child to hospital, the doctor may wish to examine the eyes as part of a routine examination. For this, he uses an ophthalmoscope which, being provided with a light and a magnifying lens, enables him to explore the fundus of the eye and to detect any abnormality of the optic disc. Thus the doctor may detect papilloedema due to the swelling of the optic nerve, indicating conditions such as brain tumour, or cerebral abscess. Further, he has the opportunity of viewing an artery directly, this being the only part of the body in which an artery is visible.

For examination of the eyes, the following will be required:

1. Ophthalmoscope with fitments, in working order.
2. Eye dropper.
3. Paper tissues.
4. Mydriatic, i.e. a substance which dilates the pupils; e.g., Mydrilate.
5. Receptacle for disposable items.

PREPARATION AND POSITION OF THE CHILD:

The examination should take place in a part of the ward which can be darkened. Whenever possible, the nurse should explain clearly to the child the steps of the procedure and warn him of the effect of the drug on his eyes. He must be told that he may see double, or that his vision may become blurred for a while. By the time the doctor arrives, the child should be adequately informed of what is going to take place and should be completely reassured. If a mydriatic has been ordered, it must be instilled thirty minutes before the examination.

Older children, where the condition permits, can be examined sitting in a chair, while infants will be examined lying on a flat surface. The nurse should hold the infant's head to restrict movement and be prepared to evert the eyelids at the doctor's direction. If the effect of the mydriatic is prolonged, eserine 0·5 per cent may be instilled to counteract this effect.

Treatments which may be carried out by the nurse include :

1. Application of ointment and eye bathing.
2. Application of heat.
3. Instillation of drops.
4. Irrigation of eyes.

1. Application of Ointment and Eye Bathing

REASONS. Ointments are applied in the following circumstances:
   (*a*) Where infection of the eyelids is present.
   (*b*) In cases of conjunctivitis to prevent the eyelids from sticking together and to allow the escape of discharge.
   (*c*) Where corneal ulcers are present or to prevent their formation.

Substances which may be used are: Albucid $2\frac{1}{2}$ per cent, chloramphenicol, penicillin, hydrocortisone, and atropine ointment.

REQUIREMENTS:

Sterile equipment :
   1. Dental rolls.
   2. Wool balls.
   3. Gallipot.
   4. Glass rod.
   5. Eye pad (see p. 146).

Additional items:

6. Warmed normal saline for bathing the eye.
7. Ointment—nearly always in nozzled tubes.
8. Receptacle for salvage.
9. Receptacle for used rods.
10. Receptacle for disposable items.

METHOD. The child is placed in a comfortable position and, provided he is old enough to understand, the procedure is explained to him. The eye is bathed from the inner to the outer aspects of the eye. The dental rolls are used for bathing the canthus and the wool balls for the eye lids and are used once only. The rod is examined carefully for any chips or cracks. It is then anointed and placed between the eyelid and the globe. The eyelid is then closed over the rod, which is rotated and then withdrawn gently.

An ointment is sometimes applied externally to the eyelids. In such a case, the ointment is gently worked into the roots of the lashes, or smeared along the lid margin with a sterile swab. Thorough cleansing of the lid margins must be carried out first.

If the ointment is in a nozzled tube, it can be squirted into the lower fornix. This requires care as the child may jump whilst the nozzle is near the eye. The nozzle must always be cleansed prior to using it.

2. Application of Heat

REASONS. The application of heat is indicated in conditions such as infected meibomian cyst, iritis and external stye. It will relieve pain and will aid in the resolution of the infection.

Heat in the form of a surgical fomentation with pad and bandage is rarely used today. Should a fomentation be ordered, the nurse must be aware of the danger of a skin burn which may lead to a spread of infection.

A more effective and less painful method of applying heat is by hot spoon bathing.

REQUIREMENTS:

1. Receiver with a small wooden spoon padded with lint.
2. Bowl of hot water, temperature 82·2°C or 180°F.
3. Gallipot with sterile swabs.

4. Lotion thermometer.

5. Receptacle for soiled swabs.

METHOD. The child is seated comfortably. The nurse explains to him what he will have to do. The spoon is immersed in the hot water and any excess water removed by pressing the spoon against the side of the bowl. The spoon is then raised to the closed eyelids without, however, touching them. This raising of the spoon to the lids is repeated every four seconds for fifteen minutes. This process may be repeated four times per day or more frequently if required.

3. Instillation of Drops

DROPS ARE INSTILLED for many purposes, some of these being:

1. To enlarge the pupils in order to facilitate examination of eyes; also in traumatic affections of the cornea, iris, and ciliary body. The drugs which may be used are atropine 1 per cent, which has a more lasting effect, or homatropine and cocaine $\frac{1}{2}$ to 1 per cent, which dilate the pupils for shorter periods.

2. To contract the pupils. Eserine 0·5 per cent is usually employed to counteract the effects of the mydriatic.

3. To counteract infection. Antibiotics such as solframycin, chloramphenicol, or chemotherapeutic agents such as albucid may be used.

Conjunctivitis, often due to staphylococcal infection, is one of the afflictions of children's eyes. In the newborn, it is known as ophthalmia neonatorum. Whenever a baby's eye is discharging, a swab must be taken and the causative organisms identified. The organism responsible may be the gonococcus which as gonococcal ophthalmia could lead to blindness. This disease is notifiable to the Public Health Authority. The infant should be isolated and intensive treatment started to prevent damage to the eyes and the possible spread of the infection.

4. To induce local anaesthesia, where a foreign body is to be removed from the cornea, opthiane 1 per cent is the drug of choice.

5. To lubricate—bland oily drops such as cod liver oil or castor oil are used in the treatment of burns or abrasions.

REQUIREMENTS:

1. Eye drops.

2. Eye dropper.

3. Paper tissues.

Additional items for bathing the eye will be required when there is conjunctivitis. See requirements for application of ointment, replacing the glass rod with an eye dropper.

METHOD. When the procedure is to be carried out on a young child or infant, two nurses should be available. It must be carried out quickly, as no child will remain still for long while a drop shimmers at the end of a dropper.

The young child or infant should be lying flat, but an older child may be in the sitting position. Holding the dropper ready, the nurse rests one hand on the child's forehead, keeping the dropper at a sufficient distance for safety in the event of a sudden jerk. With the other hand, she simultaneously draws the child's lower lid gently downwards and attracts his gaze upwards (Fig. 33). One or two drops are instilled into the lower recess of the conjunctiva and any excess which may have trickled down the cheek should be mopped up immediately.

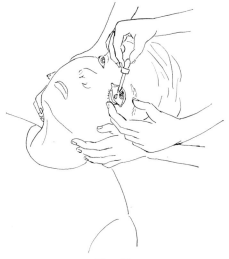

Fig. 33
Instillation of eyedrops

4. Irrigation of the Eyes

Lotions are used for cleansing the eyelids, or for irrigating the conjunctiva. They are useful in washing away fragments of mucus, foreign material, and clumps of dead cells. To avoid irritation of the conjunctiva, the lotion should be of the same concentration as lacrymal secretions; e.g., normal saline or half strength normal saline.

REQUIREMENTS:

Sterile equipment:
  1. Jug of lotion at a temperature of 37·2°C or 99°F.
  2. Lotion thermometer.
  3. Undine or eyebath.
  4. Wool balls.
  5. Large receiver.

Additional equipment:
  6. Receptacle for disposable items.
  7. Water repellent towel.

METHOD. Older children may use an eyebath, but the undine provides a more thorough irrigation. The water repellent towel is placed round the child's shoulders. The undine is filled with the lotion. The large receiver is held at the side of the face just below the eye which is to be treated. It is advisable to try the lotion on the child's cheek first to accustom him to the sensation. The flow is then directed from the inner canthus to the outer.

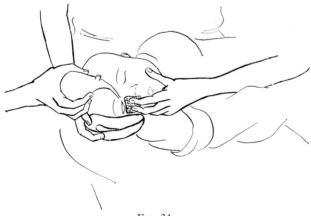

FIG. 34
Irrigation of the eye

This is in an endeavour to prevent the spread of infection to the lacrymal duct. The child should be encouraged to move his eyes freely. Finally, in the older child, the upper eyelid is everted and irrigated, but, in an infant, it is easier to pick up the upper eyelid and pull it gently away from the globe and then irrigate. It is advisable to rest the hand holding the undine on the child's forehead. The point of the undine should be held at a sufficient distance for safety in the event of a sudden jerk (Fig. 34).

When the irrigation is completed, the eyes are wiped gently, using each cotton wool ball once only.

5. Eye Pads

Eye dressings are usually not used when there is an infection of the eye, though there may be occasions when the doctor may indicate that a dressing is required. One of the reasons for applying a pad is when photophobia is present. It will also be necessary in all cases where injuries or haemorrhage of the eye has occurred.

Sterile gamgee pads are used and it may be necessary to restrain the child's arms to prevent both the removal of the pad and rubbing of the eye. If the child is distressed with the pad and it is unnecessary to omit light, then the pad may be removed.

BIBLIOGRAPHY

Forfar, U. (1961). *Aids to Ophthalmic Nursing*. London: Baillière.
Fuerst, E. V. & Wolff, L. (1964). *Fundamentals of Nursing, Eye Irrigation*. Philadelphia: Lippincott.
Garland, P. (1962). Emergency eye care. *Nurs. Times*, **58**, 435.
Harmer, B. & Henderson, V. (1955). *Principles and Practice of Nursing*, 5th ed., chap. 23. New York: Macmillan.
Hector, W. (1968). *Modern Nursing, Theory and Practice*, 4th ed., chap. 24. London: Heinemann.

CHAPTER XI

TREATMENT OF THE EAR, NOSE AND THROAT

Swabbing an ear; syringing of ears; insufflation; instillation of ear drops; examination of the nose; nasal irrigation; nasal spray; instillation of nasal drops; packing; oral hygiene.

THE EAR

THE ears are frequently the seat of much pain and discomfort in the child. This may be due to infection, sometimes to wax if it adheres to meatal skin, or to injury by foreign bodies. A nurse may be called upon to carry out several procedures, but first a few essential facts should be remembered.

The external ear consists of the pinna and external auditory meatus. In the younger child the canal is approximately one inch in length and almost straight. In the older child the canal is curved in a forward and downward direction. For examination and treatment, therefore, the pinna is gently pulled downward and backward in the young child, and upward and backward in the older child.

The middle ear is separated from the external ear by the tympanic membrane. The tympanic membrane forms an attachment with three ossicles, the malleus, incus and stapes. These are responsible, together with the tympanic membrane, for conveying sound vibrations to the inner ear. To maintain equal pressure on both sides of the tympanic membrane a small tube, the Eustachian tube, communicates with the naso-pharynx and the middle ear. This tube may become blocked through infection or catarrh, and infection may spread from the naso-pharynx along the Eustachian tube to the middle ear.

The inner ear consists of the cochlea which contains the receptors of hearing, and the semicircular canals which are concerned with the maintenance of equilibrium. Both contain fluid which is set in motion by sound vibration or movement. Heat and cold can also affect it, causing vertigo. Syringing an ear with too hot or cold a lotion will result in a severe vertigo.

Examination and Swabbing of an Ear

Swabbing may be carried out twice daily or as often as necessary. It is the method of choice for cleaning an ear when infection is present. The auditory (external) canal should be cleaned only as far as it can be seen and it is therefore necessary to have a head mirror, lamp and aural speculum. An auroscope can be used but it is more dangerous in unskilled hands, especially with a small child who may be restless and difficult to hold.

The hand that is holding the speculum should rest against the child's head so that the speculum will move with any sudden movement of the child thus avoiding injury. The practice of cleaning without clear vision is to be condemned.

REQUIREMENTS:

Sterile equipment :

1. Aural specula and cotton wool holder.
2. Cotton wall balls.
3. Gallipot for surgical spirit.

Additional equipment :

4. Head light or head mirror and light.
5. Receptacle for salvage.
6. Receptacle for instruments.
7. Receptacle for disposable items.

METHOD. Whenever possible the nurse must give adequate explanation to the child. He is held in a comfortable position and in the smaller child the arms will require to be restrained. A wisp of cotton wool is attached to the cotton wool holder. It should be firmly attached to prevent it coming off the applicator whilst cleaning the ear, and sufficient cotton wool must be left at the tip to prevent the applicator touching the tympanic membrane (Fig. 35).

The pinna of the ear is pulled backward in the smaller child and backward and upward in the older child, and the external canal cleaned. The last mop contains surgical spirit and is wiped around the canal. The ear is then examined.

Syringing of Ears

REASON. This is perhaps a more effective way of cleaning an

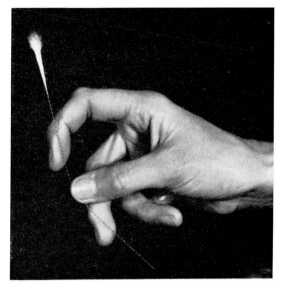

Fig. 35
Wire wool carrier, demonstrating flexibility and position
of cotton wool.

ear but is not without danger. If the treatment is for the removal
of wax, there is great danger of damage to the tympanic membrane, due to compression of the hard wax against it by introducing a jet of fluid. It could lead to perforation of the membrane
which would allow entry of organisms into the middle ear.
Injury may also be caused with the nozzle or when the fluid is
introduced with too great a force. The procedure is only carried
out on doctor's instruction.

REQUIREMENTS:

Sterile equipment :
   1. Aural syringe, speculum.
   2. Aural angled forceps.
   3. Cotton wool balls.
   4. 2 pint or 1 litre jug containing the solution at a temperature
      of 35·5-36·6°C or 96-98°F; e.g., sodium bicarbonate 4 per
      cent or normal saline.
   5. Gallipot with surgical spirit.

Additional equipment:

6. Lotion thermometer.
7. Head light or head mirror and lamp.
8. Cotton wool holder.
9. Water repellent sheet.
10. Receptacle for the returned fluid.
11. Receptacle for disposable items.
12. Receptacle for instruments.

METHOD AND CARE OF CHILD. The procedure should be explained to the older child and he should be asked to report any discomfort or nausea. The child is held in a comfortable position and a repellent sheet is placed around his shoulders. The lotion is tested with a lotion thermometer. The pinna of the ear is pulled upwards and backwards (if an older child) and, with the nozzle at the entry to the canal, the fluid is directed gently to the roof of the canal. When wax or pus has been cleared, the ear is mopped dry with surgical spirit.

If both ears require syringing, the receivers are marked left and right and the returned fluid is kept for inspection. Separate nozzles should be used and rubber tips can be fitted for additional protection.

If the wax is hard it can be softened by instilling warm olive oil 20 minutes before syringing. For very persistent wax, sodium bicarbonate solution 4 per cent or Cerumol can be instilled twice daily for three or more days before the procedure is carried out.

Insufflation of the Ear

REASON. This is a means of introducing drugs in powder form. It is carried out when infection of the external canal is present. The powder is sprayed into the canal by means of an insufflator.

REQUIREMENTS:

1. Insufflator.
2. Cotton wool holder.
3. Cotton wool balls.
4. Drug to be given; e.g., boric powder, penicillin powder, etc.
5. Receptacle for disposable items.
6. Receptacle for salvage.
7. Receptacle for instruments.

METHOD. The ear is cleaned with dry cotton wool. The insufflator is filled with the powder to be used and directed into the canal. The bulb is squeezed gently but firmly; too feeble a 'puff' may be useless.

Instillation of Ear Drops

REASONS. Drops may be instilled to soften wax, for the relief of pain or to kill insects. Substances which may be used include:
Carbolic acid 3 per cent in glycerine for the relief of pain.
Alcohol 70-90 per cent to kill insects—this may be painful because of the skin irritation the insects have caused.
Chloramphenicol 1-10 per cent in propylene glycol.

REQUIREMENTS:
1. Dropper and angled aural forceps.
2. Cotton wool balls.
3. Bottle of substance to be instilled.
4. Receptacle for instruments.
5. Receptacle for disposable items.

METHOD. Whenever possible the nurse should explain to the child what is going to be done. He should be lying down with the affected ear uppermost. The substance is slightly warmed; this can be achieved by warming the bottle or dropper in the hand. The drops are then gently inserted into the canal. The child should remain in that position for a short time till the drops are absorbed.

THE NOSE

Examination of the Nose

REASONS. This may be necessary when the child has a history of repeated colds, difficulty in breathing, persistent nasal discharge or repeated epistaxis. The nose is examined for the following:

(a) The condition of the mucous lining of the interior of the nose.
(b) The patency, i.e., the ability to breathe through one or both nostrils.
(c) The presence of discharge due to disease or irritation of the mucous membrane.
(d) Bleeding: this may be due to rupture of a capillary vessel of the nasal septum.
(e) Tenderness over the sinuses.

REQUIREMENTS:

1. Head light or head mirror and lamp.
2. Nasal specula and cotton wool carrier.
3. Cotton wool balls.
4. Receptacle for disposable articles.
5. Receptacle for instruments.

PREPARATION OF THE CHILD. The older child may sit in front of the doctor with his head slightly tilted backwards. Infants and small children should be placed on the nurse's knee, the head is supported and tilted backwards with the left hand while the nurse's right hand restrains the arms. The legs of the child are tucked between her knees.

THE NOSE MAY BE TREATED BY THE FOLLOWING MEANS:

1. Spraying.
2. Instillation of drops.
3. Packing.

Nasal Sprays

REASON. These are used for the relief of congestion, in rhinitis, and as a means of introducing a local anaesthetic. If the child is old enough (10 years of age) he may use the spray himself.

REQUIREMENTS:

Spray containing suitable substance; e.g., ephedrine 1 per cent in normal saline for congestion.

METHOD. The child is asked to sniff the substance gently as the bulb is squeezed. The spray is then held just inside one nostril and the bulb squeezed lightly.

Instillation of Nasal Drops

REASONS:

1. Used for the introduction of antibiotics to counteract inflammatory processes.
2. For the introduction of astringent drops to relieve congestion.

REQUIREMENTS:

1. Pipette with a fine piece of rubber tubing at the end.
2. Cotton wool balls.

3. Drug to be given; e.g., Otrivine.
4. Receptacle for instruments.
5. Receptacle for disposable items.

METHOD. The child is asked to blow his nose before the treatment. He is placed on his side with the head lowered. The pipette with rubber tubing is inserted just inside the nostril and the drops instilled. The child is left in this position for a few minutes and asked not to blow his nose immediately after the treatment.

Packing of the Nose

REASON. It is usually carried out to apply pressure to a bleeding point in the nose. Generally it is not done by nurses as it is difficult for them to determine where the bleeding point is. It may in fact not be in the nose, but in the posterior naso-pharynx.

Calgitex gauze is one of the preparations used. It is a sterile haemostatic preparation which when inserted into the nostril exerts pressure on the bleeding point and also produces haemostasis.

REQUIREMENTS:

1. Good light.
2. Sterile angular forceps and nasal specula.
3. Scissors and spatulae.
4. Calgitex gauze or ribbon gauze.
5. Lubricant.
6. Adhesive strapping.
7. Receptacle for instruments.
8. Receptacle for excess gauze.

METHOD. A good light and spatula will be required to examine the posterior naso-pharynx to ensure that the bleeding point does not originate from there. The gauze is inserted with the aid of angular forceps and pushed firmly into the nostril. Instead of using Calgitex, a finger cot filled with ribbon gauze or wool and dipped in glycerine, may be used. It applies pressure and does not adhere to the mucous membrane, therefore will not cause further bleeding on removal. If both nostrils are packed, the ends of the gauze are tied and secured to the face with adhesive.

To remove the Calgitex gauze it should be moistened with saline and pulled out gently.

ORAL HYGIENE

The secretions of the mouth and tonicity of the tissue may be affected quite considerably when a child is ill. In health, these tissues are kept moist and clean by the saliva secreted from the salivary glands and the secretions of the small accessory glands of the mouth. In ill health, nature does not fulfil this function on her own, and the aim of the nurse should be to complete what nature has temporarily abandoned.

To maintain the healthy state of the mouth when an infant is febrile, toxic or dehydrated, small quantities of cooled boiled water should be given to drink between feeds. Sweetened water or such substances as rose hip syrup given regularly between feeds either in sickness or in health is to be condemned; such a practice alters the composition of the secretions in the mouth and creates a medium which seriously affects the developing teeth and causes dental caries. Teeth which have not yet erupted can be affected.

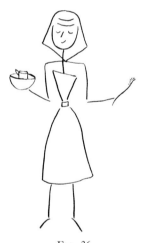

Fig. 36
Oral hygiene the natural way

Methods of Oral Hygiene

1. PHYSIOLOGICAL. Hard fibrous foods can be used to advantage after meals to remove debris from the teeth and thus assist in the

prevention of dental caries. As a normal routine, part of an apple or a carrot should be given to finish a meal when tooth brushing cannot be carried out.

2. TOOTH BRUSHING. The older child should have been taught at an early age to brush his teeth efficiently after meals. This habit must be maintained whenever possible while the child is in hospital. It should be remembered that it is the normal way of maintaining a clean and healthy mouth; it is also by far the most pleasant (Fig. 36). Even if the child is not taking solid food, a mouth wash and tooth brushing is to be preferred to swabbing the mouth with a variety of lotions. Tooth brushing should be methodical. Brush the teeth from the gum margin to the tooth surface and along the biting surfaces. Effective tooth brushing takes four minutes. The tooth brush should be of medium hardness, either nylon or bristle, and be hung separately to dry after use. It is preferable to have tooth paste from a tube, which has a screw cap, rather than from a tin which may be left open and used by several people rubbing their brush on the compressed cake. Tooth brushing should be supervised up to the age of approximately six years.

3. SIALOGOGUE. Salivary stimulant.
Action: Stimulating and refreshing.
Method : Lemon drops can be used for stimulating salivary flow.
Indication: Maintenance of a clean mouth; e.g., (i) febrile child with diminished supply of saliva, and (ii) after major orthodontic surgery when the child is unable to open his mouth sufficiently for other means of cleansing.

4. RINSES.
Action: Mechanical. Rinses are used to remove debris after tooth brushing.
Lotions: Water or normal saline.

5. MOUTH WASHES. Mouth washes are used before, or in place of other methods of cleansing to loosen the debris from between the teeth. The lotion should be swilled round the mouth and forced several times against the teeth before spitting out into a bowl. This habit is now being taught in schools and is routinely carried out after meals. Plain water can be used.

Lotions for Mouth Washes and Irrigations

A variety of lotions exist and it is essential that there should be an understanding of action and use.

(i) SODIUM PERBORATE: Trade name Bocasan.

Action : Cleansing and active against anaerobic organisms.

Strength : Dissolve one packet of powder in the prescribed amount of water.

Method : Mouth wash. The child must hold the fluid in his mouth for one and a half minutes. If this creates a difficulty, it can be achieved by asking him to suck a dental roll saturated in the solution, or by placing the dental roll just inside the cheek alongside the gums.

Sodium perborate is effective while nascent oxygen is released. It is this effervescent action that is important and it is, therefore, of little value to use the solution unless it can be retained in the mouth for the recommended length of time.

Indications—Infected mouth.

Contra-indications—This substance should not be used where there is an open wound as it can drive infection into the raw surface.

(ii) HYDROGEN PEROXIDE 10 VOLUMES.

Action : Cleansing and active against anaerobic organisms.

Strength : One teaspoonful of 10 volumes to 5 ounces of water.

Method, Indications and Contra-indications are as for sodium perborate.

(iii) BICARBONATE OF SODA.

Action : Cleansing and fat solvent.

Strength : One rounded teaspoonful of the powder to 10 ounces of water.

Method : Mouth wash, swabbing the mouth, or as an irrigation.

Indications : (*a*) following surgery four hours after all evidence of haemorrhage has ceased, and (*b*) neglected mouth.

(iv) HYPERTONIC SALINE.

Action : Astringent.

Strength : One teaspoonful sodium chloride to 10 ounces of water.

Method : Mouth wash, swabbing the mouth, or as an irrigation.

Indications : Following surgery or traumatic injury.

(v) PHENOL SODIQUE.

   Action : Mechanical cleanser.

   Strength : ½ ounce concentrate to 5 ounces of water.

   Method : Mouth wash, swabbing the mouth, or irrigation.

   Indications : (*a*) Cleansing and maintaining a healthy mouth,
   (*b*) neglected mouth.

(vi) GLYCOTHYMOLINE.

   Action : Refreshing, mildly bacteriostatic, bacteriocidal.

   Strength : One ounce of concentrate to five ounces of water.

   Method : Mouth wash, swabbing the mouth.

   Indications : Maintenance of a healthy mouth.

   Soluble effervescent tablets containing thymoline are also
available. One tablet dissolved in half a tumbler of warm water
provides an effective mouth wash for older children.

   Tap water is adequate for making the solutions unless surgery
has been carried out when sterile water and sterile equipment
should be used.

Swabbing the Mouth

   When the child is unable to brush his teeth, special treatment
of the mouth will have to be carried out. A tray should be prepared
and care given two- or four-hourly when the child is awake.

REQUIREMENTS:

1. 1 pr. dissecting forceps.
2. 1 pr. small swab holding forceps or artery forceps.
3. Small swabs and dental rolls.
4. Lotions for use with required number of gallipots.
5. Petroleum jelly or lanoline.
6. Box of paper tissues.
7. Receptacle for instruments.
8. Receptacle for disposable items.

METHOD. A paper tissue is placed under the child's chin. The
lips are smeared with petroleum jelly to prevent lotions entering
cracks and causing unnecessary pain. The mouth is gently opened
and the inside of the cheeks, the teeth, all crevices around the gums,
the roof of the mouth, and the tongue swabbed.

   A dressed pair of forceps is used, care being taken to ensure
that the forceps is covered and does not scratch or injure the child

in any way. The use of artery forceps for infants is helpful; by clamping the swab or dental roll, there is no fear of either being lost or inadvertently swallowed. After swabbing, the lips are dried and again smeared with petroleum jelly.

Cracked lips provide a portal of entry for organisms and it is, therefore, important to keep them lubricated.

Irrigation of the Mouth

This may be the method of choice when the child is unable to open his mouth adequately for other cleansing, or when trauma or infection leaves an unhealed surface.

REQUIREMENTS:

Sterile equipment :
1. Chip syringe, or Higginson syringe with a fine catheter No. 10 F.G. or 4 E.G.
2. Jug containing lotion.
3. Bowl of warm water to heat lotion.
4. Lotion thermometer.
5. Lubrication for lips.

Additional equipment :
6. Mackintosh cape.
7. Box of paper tissues.
8. Paper towels.
9. Receiver for used lotion.
10. Receptacle for disposable items.

METHOD. The child is protected with a mackintosh and a paper towel is tucked under his chin. The lotion is tested and the syringe filled. It is then gently introduced into the mouth. The flow of lotion should be directed from behind forwards, so that it flows over the surface of the wound, but is not directed into it.

LESIONS OF THE MOUTH AND THROAT

Those which occur frequently in children are caused by: (i) fungi, (ii) ulceration, and (iii) trauma with or without infection. The organisms which are found most frequently are the Haemolytic Streptococcus and the Candida or Monilia albicans. The areas infected include the gingiva, gum margins, buccal mucous membrane, tongue, tonsils, pharynx and larynx, leading to conditions such as gingivitis, fungus infections, tonsillitis, pharyngitis, laryngitis and laryngeal stridor or quinsy.

Some Specific Therapeutic Methods of Treatment
Application of aqueous solution of Gentian Violet ½ per cent

The solution must be freshly prepared because evaporation and decomposition occur and if applied could lead to ulceration of the mucous membrane.

METHOD. Sterile water should be given after a milk feed or meal, the lips are then lubricated with petroleum jelly and two drops of the solution dropped on to the tongue. It is then spread to every area of the mouth and throat by means of the saliva. The petroleum jelly prevents staining of the lips.

Local antibiotics are given by the same method.

Nystatin, which is used widely on Monilia infections, if kept at room temperature remains active for seven days once it has been reconstituted. Other drugs may have even shorter periods of activity and it is essential to read the accompanying literature. Local applications to the mouth are always carried out for a limited period. Prolonged application can lead to ulceration and severe complications. The customary period of time for an application of the drug is four times per day over a period of three days. Forty-eight hours later, a mouth swab is taken and sent for culture of micro-organisms, but directions should be issued by the medical staff.

Crusts around the lips should not be separated forcibly as once removed a raw surface remains which constitutes a further portal of entry for infection.

Small children and infants require arm splints when any infection of the mouth exists. Finger sucking and picking crusts delays healing and spreads infection. Woollen garments, which cannot be laundered, should be avoided as they provide a grave source of infection.

Gargles

These are excellent for cleansing and soothing purposes, but can only be given effectively to children of seven years of age and upwards. The solution should be warm and the lotions given for mouth washes can all be used for gargling.

Application of 10 per cent Chromic Acid

This may be ordered to be applied to ulcer craters of the mouth to relieve pain. It is essential to have the child's confidence and to ensure he will keep his mouth open during the process. Craters should be lightly touched once with a dressed probe. The tip of the cotton wool only should be dipped into the solution to avoid dripping any on the inside of the mouth.

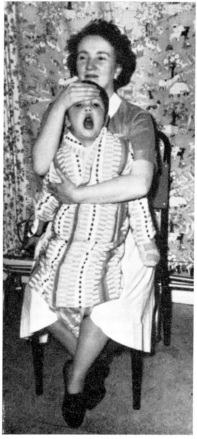

Fig. 37
Child being held for examination of the throat.

Examination of the Mouth and Throat

REQUIREMENTS:
1. Head light or head mirror and lamp.
2. Tray with:
    (a) Tongue depresser.
    (b) Post nasal mirror.
    (c) Laryngeal mirrors, curved and straight.
    (d) Fine dissecting forceps.
    (e) Dental rolls.
    (f) Throat swabs.
3. Box of paper tissues.
4. Receptacle for paper tissues.
5. Receptacle for used instruments.

PREPARATION OF THE CHILD. The small child should be sitting on the nurse's knee, facing the doctor, with head tilted back and supported. The child's legs may be held between the nurse's knees. It is essential to reassure and calm the child before examination begins (Fig. 37).

BIBLIOGRAPHY

Birrell, J. F. (1961). *The Ear, Nose and Throat Diseases of Children*. London: Cassell.
Markham, J. (1962). Care of the mouth. *Nurs. Times*, **58**, 1385.
Marshall, S. (1967). *Aids to Ear, Nose and Throat Nursing*, 4th ed. London: Baillière.

G

CHAPTER XII

PROCEDURES RELATING TO THE RESPIRATORY SYSTEM

Administration of oxygen; bronchoscopy; tracheostomy; naso-tracheal intubation; positive pressure ventilation; mucolytic agents; underwater seal drainage.

ADMINISTRATION OF OXYGEN

OXYGEN is a colourless, odourless and tasteless gas. Tissue cells must be constantly supplied with oxygen, therefore oxygen inhalation is essential for life. In certain circumstances deficiency of oxygen may occur. The nurse has the greatest opportunity to observe signs of hypoxia and early recognition of these signs is essential.

Some of these include: rapid and shallow breathing, cyanosis, increased restlessness and an increase in pulse rate. Measurement of the blood gases is an important factor in differential diagnosis of hypoxia. The Astrup technique is employed to determine pO_2, pCO_2 and pH, i.e., tension of oxygen and carbon dioxide in the blood and hydrogen ion concentration.

Indications for Oxygen Therapy

A. *Disorders of the respiratory or cardio-vascular system* where there is interference with the transfer of oxygen from inspired air to the haemoglobin:

1. Respiratory centre depression—excessive morphine or barbiturates; raised intra-cranial pressure, etc.
2. Respiratory tract obstructions:
   (*a*) upper respiratory tract—acute laryngo-tracheo-bronchitis.
   (*b*) lower respiratory tract—e.g., asthma.
3. Acute lower respiratory tract infections.
4. Chronic respiratory insufficiency—e.g., cystic fibrosis.
5. Pulmonary oedema—as in cardiac failure.

B. *Disorders in which the oxygen-carrying ability of the blood is decreased:*

   1. Severe anaemia.

   2. Carbon monoxide poisoning.

C. *Conditions in which the circulation is slowed ·*

   1. Cardiac failure.

   2. Shock—septicaemia, trauma, dehydration.

D. *Conditions in which tissues are unable to utilise oxygen*—e.g., cyanide poisoning.

Methods of Administration of Oxygen

Several methods may be employed; the one of choice is dependent on the age of the child and is the one which will give an adequate concentration of oxygen with the least disturbance to the child. In all methods some means of humidification is essential as without it, oxygen can be an irritant in the alveoli, stimulating the production of mucus.

The Oxygen Tent

The concentration of oxygen within the tent will depend on the efficiency of the tent and the rate of flow of oxygen, but a concentration of 50-60 per cent can be produced, with a flow of oxygen of 6-8 litres per minute achieving 50 per cent concentration (Humidaire tent—Oxygenaire—Simpson and Russell).

The back chamber containing ice keeps the atmosphere cool and moist though it does not create a high humidity. The temperature within the tent should be recorded frequently and a temperature of 17·7-21·1°C or 64-70°F maintained. The tent is placed over the bed and tucked in all round. Nursing procedures are carried out through pockets or sleeves. Flushing of the tent is necessary after the sides have been opened. This should be carried out according to the manufacturer's instructions. Twenty litres per minute for 20 minutes is necessary for the Humidaire.

It is important to check the oxygen concentration in a tent or incubator. A simple method is by the use of the MIRA analyser (Chapter IV). Recent studies carried out at the Royal Hospital for Sick Children, Edinburgh (Simpson and Russell), demonstrate that incubators generally achieved the concentrations claimed for them, but that tents could be considerably below specification.

The Incubator (see Chapter IV)

This is ideal for the infant in the neonatal period.

By Disposable Polythene Mask

Emergency administration of oxygen can be given with the use of a disposable face mask which covers the mouth and nose but not the eyes. These are packed in cellophane bags and supplied in three sizes. They are useful for infants and children over 4 years of age. The smaller child does not generally tolerate anything over the face (Fig. 38).

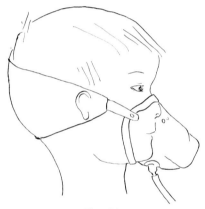

Fig. 38
Disposable oxygen mask

METHOD. The treatment should be explained to the child and his co-operation obtained. A mask of suitable size should be selected. The oxygen is turned on at a slightly higher rate of flow than will be required. The mask is then adjusted so that it fits snugly over the child's face. This can be achieved by moulding the malleable wire and adjusting the elastic. It is important to ensure that the oxygen is not being blown into the child's eyes. The flow of oxygen is then adjusted to the required rate. The oxygen within the mask is kept at a suitable humidity by the deposit of moisture from the air exhaled by the child.

When no disposable mask is available, a funnel may be used in an emergency. This is held one to two inches from the face. This method is very wasteful and not very effective.

Nasal Catheter

This method is of use when a child cannot tolerate a mask and it is undesirable to have the child in an oxygen tent; e.g., the child with extensive burns.

The nostrils are cleaned. The catheter is connected to the oxygen supply and the flow commenced. The catheter is passed gently into the naso-pharynx, and fixed to the cheek. A transfer bottle is used to pass oxygen through water to humidify the oxygen. The oxygen is turned on before the catheter is inserted to prevent the traumatic effect of a sudden release of pressure. The rate of flow must be adjusted as ordered. If oxygen is to be administered for any length of time, a Y-connection can be incorporated in the tubing to ensure that the concentration of oxygen given is not too high. Pressure tubing must be used.

Perspex Cot Cover

This is useful for infants lying in a Sorrento or Belfast cot. The oxygen is piped into the cot through a small hole. An accurate flowmeter should be used and the concentration of oxygen within the cot analysed at frequent intervals (analysis of oxygen concentration, Chapter IV). The temperature of the atmosphere should be recorded and, if necessary, a small bowl containing ice can be placed in a safe position in the cot to keep the atmosphere cool.

When oxygen is being administered, it is important to use the correct anti-static pressure tubing. This will not collapse or become kinked, thus inadvertently cutting off the oxygen supply.

Points to note

Grease or oil should not be allowed to come in contact with the pressure gauge or the oxygen cylinder as this could precipitate an explosion and fire when oxygen is released. A flowmeter and fine adjustment valve are attached to each cylinder and when changing cylinders it is necessary to tighten these only sufficiently to avoid leakage. Unnecessary hammering will only damage the valve. Used cylinders should be clearly marked 'empty' and kept in a separate area.

Visitors to children must be warned not to smoke or light a

match as combustion will occur much more readily in the presence of oxygen, leading to serious fires. Mechanical toys which spark must also not be used for this reason.

BRONCHOSCOPY

This is a direct vision examination of the trachea and the main bronchial tubes. It is not only an aid to diagnosis, but also a means of access to the lower reaches of the trachea and the main bronchi for biopsy and for the removal of foreign bodies in these structures.

PREPARATION FOR THE PROCEDURE. Special bronchoscopes of varying sizes are used with suckers, or long biopsy forceps. The bronchoscopes contain light carriers. Sterilisation of the light carriers and flex can be carried out by immersion in biniodide of mercury 1:5000 for fifteen minutes, or by using a formalin cabinet. Flex which is not rubber backed or covered with plastic can only be wiped with a disinfectant. A powerful sucker with adequate length of rubber tubing from the suction bottle is essential. The bottle contains approximately two inches of water —this is merely to facilitate cleaning of the bottle. Instruments and batteries must be tested and in working order. A bowl of sterile water is placed near the suckers for rinsing purposes. A specimen bottle may be attached to the equipment by means of a disposable sterile unit which fits on to a universal container. Such units are supplied pre-sterilised by Oxygenaire (London) Ltd.

REQUIREMENTS:

Trolley with sterile equipment on upper shelf:
  1. Laryngoscope and three blades.
  2. Bronchoscopes (size according to the doctor's instructions).
  3. Light carriers to match bronchoscopes, with bulbs.
  4. Two crocodile forceps.
  5. Foreign body and biopsy forceps.
  6. Three to four suckers.
  7. Swabs.
  8. Specimen jar to attach to the suction apparatus.

Lower shelf:
  1. Battery box with leads.
  2. Receptacle for disposable items.

Additional items :

Equipment for the administration of an anaesthetic.

Resuscitation equipment (Chapter XX).

PREPARATION OF THE CHILD. This procedure is carried out under general anaesthetic. The child is therefore prepared for a general anaesthetic and dressed in a jacket with front opening. Premedication is given prior to the procedure, the drug, dose and time being in accordance with the doctor's instructions. The child is placed on the table, his head extended so that the trachea is in a straight line, and his arms placed straight at the sides, resting below each buttock. He is covered with a cotton blanket to avoid fluff.

AFTER CARE OF THE CHILD. This examination may result in serious complications and it is, therefore, essential that the nurse should watch for any signs of difficulty in breathing and summon medical aid at once. Respiratory obstruction may occur due to oedema of the lax subglottic tissue of the infant under two or three years of age. It is much less likely to occur in the older child. The anaesthetist may have to introduce an endotracheal tube or in extreme cases, if the respiratory embarrassment is severe, a tracheostomy may be performed to provide an air entry to the lungs.

After the examination and while the child is unconscious, he is nursed in the lateral, head low position to ensure drainage of mucus and saliva which otherwise may irritate the lung tissue. Suction may be required, and used when necessary to clear the pharynx. The catheter must be passed into the secretions only as far as it can be seen to avoid danger of trauma to the mucous membranes (Chapter XX).

Until the effects of general anaesthesia have abated and the cough and swallowing reflexes have returned, the child must be watched carefully. When consciousness has returned, the child is changed gradually to the upright position and encouraged in deep breathing. When the cough and swallowing reflexes have returned, fluids may be given slowly in small quantities.

A Croupette, Humidaire, or other apparatus may be used to create a humid atmosphere for the young child if respiratory distress is present following bronchoscopy.

A difficult bronchoscopy may cause trauma to the mucous lining of the bronchi leading to inflammation and pneumonia.

TRACHEOSTOMY

The operation of tracheostomy is performed for the relief of an airway which has become obstructed, or is in danger of becoming obstructed, at or above the level of the subglottic area. There are a number of conditions when this danger is a grave possibility. The most common of those are the acute inflammatory conditions causing oedema of the larynx as in laryngo-tracheo-bronchitis. An inhaled foreign body, or a scald from inhaled steam, may also give rise to oedema of the larynx and increasing respiratory obstruction. A small diamond shaped or circular opening (os) is made in the trachea, hence the name 'tracheostomy'. A tracheostomy tube is inserted into the opening.

Tracheostomy is a life saving measure; so also is the after care of the child, which requires great vigilance and care in the maintenance of a clear airway. The child should not be left alone and the period of time for which he requires an individual nurse is dependent upon his condition and progress.

TRACHEOSTOMY TUBES

A polyvinyl chloride tube may be used. This is a single tube, which is pliable, non-irritant and has been found suitable for small infants. It is satisfactory for prolonged use. The tube is secured with tape at the back of the neck and no dressing is required.

A *silver tracheostomy* tube consists of an inner and outer tube. The inner tube is removed for cleansing; it is slightly longer than the outer tube. Initially, it is not tied or clipped in position to facilitate urgent clearing of the airway. The outer tube is firmly tied with tape at the back of the neck.

PREPARATION OF THE CHILD. Preparation of the child is as for anaesthesia, and if he is old enough and sufficiently fit, some explanation as to the relief he will obtain from a different way of breathing will be reassuring.

REQUIREMENTS FOR AFTER CARE:

Sterile equipment for cleansing the tube and clearing the airway :

1. Gauze swabs, pipe cleaners for silver tube.
2. Container with saturated solution of sodium bicarbonate or normal saline.
3. 2 prs. dissecting forceps or disposable gloves.

4. Catheter for suction.
5. Suction apparatus.
6. Bowl of water for clearing catheters.
7. Receptacle for disposable items.

Separate tray with sterile equipment for renewing dressing if required :
1. Keyhole dressing and small swabs.
2. Container for cleansing lotion.
3. 2 prs. dressing forceps.

For emergency use only :
Sealed sterilised packet containing:
1. Spare tracheostomy tube and introducer.
2. Fine catheter.
3. Tracheal dilators.

The tracheostomy tube must be identical in size and type to the one in use. The catheter can be used to act as a guide should there be difficulty in introducing the tube. The catheter is threaded through the tracheostomy tube and passed into the opening down the trachea. The tube is then guided into position.

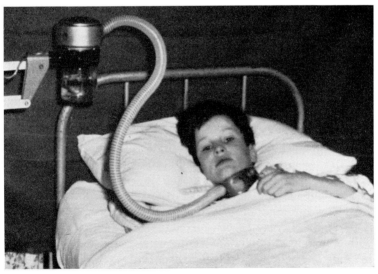

Fig. 39
Hydrojette with tracheostomy collar

Additional Requirements:

1. Humidifier. Type according to age of the child and equipment available—Croupette, Croupaire, Hydrojette, Humidaire (Fig. 39).
2. Arm restraints as necessary.
3. Requirements for oral hygiene.
4. Equipment for bronchoscopy for emergency or routine use may be required when secretions are excessive.

AFTER CARE OF THE CHILD. A great deal of the success of the after care of a child with a tracheostomy depends upon the attitude of the nurse and on her ability to comfort and reassure the child in a very frightening situation. A frightened child produces an increased amount of mucus, causing more distress and further endangering the airway. It is, therefore, essential that the nurse is able to give a feeling of confidence and can act calmly in an emergency.

The routine care to be given will vary according to the reason for the tracheostomy. When no infection is present, the use of suction may not be necessary. Medical orders must be carried out carefully and with intelligent understanding of the needs of the child. Unnecessary fear, discomfort, and trauma can result from inexpert use of suction. Trauma of the mucosa of the trachea or bronchi will cause haemorrhage, thereby greatly endangering the child's life. It is, therefore, essential that all members of the team caring for a child with a tracheostomy understand how to maintain a clear airway, and the exact procedure to be followed when suction is used. It is important that each nurse knows and can recognise early signs of respiratory obstruction and can act efficiently and effectively when it occurs.

POSITION. The semi-upright position is usually most comfortable and the one in which the child can most easily breathe.

The infant presents a rather greater nursing problem. The neck is short and all too easily the head may fall forward, occluding the airway. Positioning of such infants is, therefore, of the utmost importance. It may be considered safer to nurse the infant flat with a small firm pillow under the neck and shoulders with the head of the bed elevated, but the difficulty of maintaining this position is obvious and requires the constant attention of the nurse. Small arm splints are a necessity for the younger child until he is accustomed to the tube and will not pull it out. These should be applied immediately before or after the operation.

THE CARE AND CLEANSING OF THE AIRWAY. The method of cleansing may vary but the following important points apply to all methods:

1. Clearing must be adequate to maintain a good airway and skill is necessary to avoid injury to the child.

2. Equipment used must be sterile and care taken to prevent the introduction of micro-organisms.

3. When silver tubes are used, the inner tube is replaced inside the outer tube as soon as the airway is cleared.

4. No material is used which would cause irritation to the trachea, such as dry cotton wool.

SUGGESTED METHOD OF MAINTAINING A CLEAR AIRWAY. The hands are washed and dried. If a silver tube is used, it is removed and immersed in sodium bicarbonate. Forceps or a gloved hand are used to pass the catheter into the tracheostomy opening beyond the level of the tube; the distance required should be decided beforehand. Once in position, the suction is turned on and the catheter gradually withdrawn. It must never be left in one position. By gradually withdrawing it, air can enter past the catheter into the lungs. The vacuum of the suction apparatus is 25 cm. Hg or 10 inches Hg. The catheter must never block the tracheostomy tube completely and suction should not be applied for longer than the breath can be held. Excessive suction can completely block off a segment of lung causing it to collapse by withdrawing the residual air. Oxygen should be given directly to the tracheostomy tube for a brief period if the catheter requires to be inserted three times in succession. The use of a whistle tip catheter for suction with two lateral holes is an added safeguard against injury to the mucosa.

A straight catheter will invariably enter the right bronchus. If it is necessary to clear the left bronchus, this may be done by using an angled or Tieman's catheter No. 3 F.G. The ability to clear the airway adequately is an essential part of the nursing care and requires skill and extreme caution. It may be necessary to instil 2 ml. normal saline into the tracheostomy tube hourly prior to suction, to ensure that secretions do not become encrusted.

The inner tube is thoroughly cleansed and replaced. The area around the tube is cleansed as necessary. Catheters used for suction should be used on one occasion only because of the grave risk of introducing infected substances into the lung. Naso-pharyngeal suction may also be necessary. A separate catheter must be used and great care taken not to cause injury to the mucosa. The catheter should be inserted into the secretions and the suction turned on, gradually withdrawing the catheter and repeating the procedure if necessary.

ATMOSPHERE. Inspired air has no natural way of being warmed and moistened when the nasal passages are by-passed. The air we breathe normally contains water vapour in varying amounts, dependent on the prevailing climatic conditions. There is a danger of blockage due to dried secretions and to avoid this, a humidifier should be used to moisten the inspired air. Similarly, if oxygen administration is necessary it is essential to pass it through a humidifier to prevent crusting and hence blockage. For at least the first twenty-four hours, these children are best nursed in a moist atmosphere (Fig. 39).

ORAL HYGIENE. Oral hygiene is important in an endeavour to minimise infection. The method is dependent on the condition of the child (Chapter XI).

SPEECH. The voice will not function normally and though children are very quick to adapt and learn to speak again this will not be for at least several days. It is, therefore, important that the older child understands the position and is given pencil and paper to communicate with as soon as he is well enough.

Removal of the Tube

The child, once he has recovered from his illness, quickly adapts to the tracheostomy and may well be very apprehensive when the time comes to discard it. This period requires much patience and persuasion on the part of the nurse and her understanding is of inestimable value in adapting the child to further changes and in helping him to overcome his very natural fears. The tube may be removed under anaesthesia, or occluded for an increasing period of time daily until it is finally removed allowing the wound to close itself.

NASO-TRACHEAL INTUBATION WITH POSITIVE PRESSURE VENTILATION

The use of naso-tracheal intubation as an alternative to tracheostomy has proved of value in the care of small children and infants. With this method, there is less difficulty in maintaining a clear airway as the problems of keeping the infant in a position which will not obstruct the tracheostomy are considerable.

Naso-tracheal intubation may be used as a means of providing prolonged intermittent positive pressure ventilation of the lungs.

The Jackson Rees catheter (Fig. 40) has been found to be a safe and reliable tube when ventilation is required.

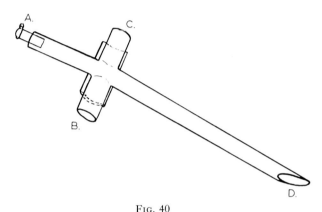

FIG. 40

Jackson Rees catheter

A. Suction limb
B and C. Inspiratory and expiratory cross-pieces
D. Tip of catheter

The inspiratory and expiratory cross-pieces B and C are attached to the positive pressure ventilator by the anaesthetist and the whole is immobilised with a head harness. A sterile spigot is inserted into the suction limb A.

The infant requires constant nursing care. No clothing should cover the chest as any change in chest movement may be the first indication of difficulty. Restlessness and a rising pulse are also danger signs.

Any deterioration in the chest movement, coupled with a progressive increase on the ventilator pressure dial, are signs of impending obstruction of the lumen of the catheter and require immediate action. Moist sounds on inspiration or expiration may also give warning, but need not necessarily be present.

The common cause of obstruction is dried secretions adherent to the tube.

On the first sign of obstruction, ventilation is discontinued, the spigot removed from the suction limb, and 2-4 ml. sterile 0·9 per cent saline should be slowly run in through a sterile suction catheter placed in the suction limb. The catheter is then attached to the suction machine giving a negative pressure of 15-20 mm. Hg, and the catheter slowly withdrawn. If, after three attempts, the lumen is not clear, medical help should be sought and re-intubation undertaken. The suction catheter should be passed only just beyond the tip of the Jackson Rees catheter (point D, Fig. 40). It must never be kept stationary, but be gradually withdrawn as suction is applied. Collapse of the lung will occur with excessive suction. A spare catheter suitably marked can act as a guide to the length the catheter is to be inserted.

It is essential that all precautions are taken to avoid transmission of infection to the infant. An aseptic technique is used. Sterile disposable polyvinyl catheters have been found to be most suitable.

Care must be taken when nursing children with a Jackson Rees catheter in position that occlusion at the cross-piece does not occur. This can happen if limbs B and C are not maintained in a position following the contours of the face. Excess padding under either limb can contribute to this.

MECHANICAL VENTILATION is used as a means of maintaining life when normal respiratory effort is inadequate. It is used as a means of eliminating carbon dioxide. There are many types of ventilators in use and there is adequate literature supplied with each one of them. It is important that the nurse has a working knowledge of the respirator in use. The anaesthetist will lay down clear guiding lines for its use.

It should not be forgotten that among the machinery is a child, who is not only alive but, if conscious, will be very frightened. It is essential that the nurse understands the importance of observation of the person, and not merely of the machine.

Control of adequate humidity is vital in the prevention of hard crusts, resulting in obstruction. Directions must be carefully followed as there are dangers of overloading the circulation of the young infant who is nursed continuously in a high humidity.

MUCOLYTIC AGENTS

These are substances which reduce the viscosity of secretions by direct action in the bronchial lumen. Their use is important in such conditions as fibrocystic disease of the pancreas where there is thick tenacious mucus, and there may be a superimposed infection with thick purulent secretions.

In the most simple form it can be given as an aerosol by methods already described. The most penetrating mist can be obtained from an ultrasonic nebuliser.

Various chemical agents have been produced which alter secretions chemically. Acetylcysteine (Airbron) has been found effective. It may be given by nebulisation or by instillation. Detergent inhalations such as Alivaire can be used as aerosols.

CHEST ASPIRATION

REASONS. This procedure is carried out for diagnostic purposes to obtain a specimen of pus or serous fluid for examination, or as a therapeutic measure to relieve pressure within the pleural cavity caused by air (a pneumothorax), blood (a haemothorax), purulent fluid (pyothorax), or a combination of these conditions.

REQUIREMENTS:

Sterile equipment :

1. Skin cleansing requisites.
2. Swabs.
3. Tray with:
   (*a*) selection of wide-bore needles with short bevels.
   (*b*) two-way syringe or 20 ml. syringe with a two-way tap.
   (*c*) rubber tubing to fit the two-way tap.
4. 2 ml. syringe and hypodermic needles for local anaesthesia.
5. Receptacle for excess fluid.
6. 2 specimen tubes:
   (*a*) for bacteriological examination, a plain tube.
   (*b*) for cytological examination, oxalate tube.

Additional equipment :

7. Antibiotics and ampoules of sterile water.
8. File.
9. Receptacle for salvage.
10. Receptacle for instruments.
11. Receptacle for disposable items.

PREPARATION OF THE CHILD. If possible, explain to the child what is happening. He will require to be kept very still and avoid coughing during the procedure. The nurse looking after him places him in the position requested by the doctor. If the child is in the sitting position, the shoulders should be raised by the nurse to the hunched position. This will increase the intercostal space, thereby making the procedure easier.

Infants are placed across a pillow, the affected side uppermost. Here the nurse increases the intercostal space by raising the shoulder and arm of that side.

It must be appreciated that this procedure may lead to respiratory distress. The nurse must, therefore, watch the child carefully and report any change to the doctor immediately. Means of resuscitation must be readily available (Chapter XX).

AFTER CARE OF THE CHILD. After the procedure, the child is moved gently into a comfortable position. The pulse and respiration rate are recorded and the child should not be left alone until the nurse is confident that there is no respiratory distress. Discomfort felt at the time of aspiration should be temporary and the respiratory distress should markedly decrease after the procedure. Any recurrence of distress must be reported immediately.

The specimen is labelled clearly and sent to the appropriate department.

UNDER WATER SEAL DRAINAGE

The management and principles involved will be better understood if the mechanics of respiration are briefly considered.

The chest cavity is an airtight compartment with movable walls. Suspended in this compartment are the lungs which communicate with the atmosphere via the trachea and the bronchi. The outer surface of the lungs is covered by a delicate serous membrane, the visceral pleura. As the main bronchus enters the lung, the membrane doubles back to become the parietal pleura. The parietal pleura lines the inner surface of the thoracic walls and the upper surface of the diaphragm. These two membranes are separated by a thin film of serous fluid and the potential space between them is known as the pleural cavity.

The pressure within the lungs is that of the atmosphere. If the lungs were solid this pressure would be transmitted to the walls of the thorax, but the lungs are elastic and the elastic recoil of the lungs tends to separate the parietal and visceral pleura, so that the pressure within the pleural cavity is at all times less than that of the atmosphere. Such pressure is called negative pressure.

On inspiration, outward movement of the chest walls enlarges the thorax. The lungs follow this movement, expanding and increasing their recoil force as air is drawn in. The intrapleural pressure, already negative, becomes increasingly negative at this point. Expiration then takes place as the recoil of the elastic tissues occurs and the rib cage and diaphragm return to their position of rest.

If the pleural cavity is opened to the atmosphere, the negative intrapleural pressure will cease to exist. The pressure outside and inside the lung will be the same and, therefore, the lung cannot expand. The elasticity of the lung tissue will cause it to collapse. This occurs when the pleural cavity is opened into traumatically, or surgically, where a drainage tube is inserted between the pleural layers. When drainage of the cavity is necessary, under water seal drainage is used. The seal prevents the entry of air but, at the same time, permits expansion of the lungs. The extent of the pneumothorax is reduced by the escape of air, and blood or exudate can be drained.

PLEURAL DRAINAGE is undertaken for the following reasons:

1. Routinely after operation on the chest to prevent a tension pneumothorax, (a) when lung tissue has been cut and air from the cut surface may continue to leak, (b) to facilitate drainage when a large raw area has been left and continual oozing of blood in the post-operative period is to be expected, and (c) to facilitate drainage when the oesophagus has been opened and there is possible contamination or leakage from the suture line.

2. To facilitate drainage after injury when haemothorax or pneumothorax is present.

3. To relieve a tension pneumothorax following a spontaneous pneumothorax, i.e. after rupture of a lung bulla.

4. To relieve an empyema.

Under Water Seal Drainage Apparatus

REQUIREMENTS. Previously sterilised and tested to ensure a secure fit.

1. Bottle with 2 holed fitting cork.
2. Length of right angled glass tubing approximately 5 inches.
3. Length of glass tubing approximately 3 inches longer than the bottle with the cork.
4. Tubing, length from the floor to the patient, optimum 100 cm.
5. Connection.
6. Sterile distilled water.

Adhesive strapping and safety pin.

METHOD. The apparatus is assembled as in the diagram with the long glass tube approximately 3 cm. or $1\frac{1}{2}$ in. under the surface of the water. The surgeon inserts the self-retaining catheter in the most dependent part of the cavity where exudate will collect. The catheter is kept firmly clamped until it is fixed to the apparatus. When the clamps are released, blood and exudate will flow by gravity through the tube to the bottle. The glass tubing below the surface of the water forms a one way valve that permits air to be forced out of the cavity by the more positive (though never actually positive) pressure developed during expiration and prevents air being taken in during inspiration. This is confirmed by bubbles escaping through the water during expiration and the column rising in the tube during inspiration. As the lung expands, the vacuum created draws the fluid only a short way up the glass tube in the bottle (Fig. 41). When the lung occupies the whole of the hemithorax the difference in pressure in the pleural cavity between inspiration and expiration is small and the oscillation in the tube may be only about 2 cm. If, however, there is atelectasis with poor or non-expansion of the lung, the lung fails to fill the space designed for it, and large fluctuations in pressure in the pleural cavity will occur on breathing, there will be a corresponding increase in the oscillations observed in the glass tube. The greater the height of the oscillation, the poorer the expansion of the lung. The height between the chest and the surface of the water seal should be sufficient to prevent water being drawn into the chest by maximum inspiratory effort. A strong inspiratory effort may produce a negative pressure equal to a 60 cm. column of water. Therefore, a height of 100 cm. is advisable.

Occasionally, suction may be applied but this is only carried out on medical orders because of the dangers involved.

Important Factors:

1. Should the suction be too powerful, the resultant negative pressure would make expiration impossible.
2. Suction encourages bleeding.
3. Suction may attract the lung to the catheter.

NURSING CARE OF THE CHILD. Careful positioning of the child is important, so that there is no pull on the tubing and so that the child does not compress it in any way. Adhesive tape can be attached to the tubing and pinned to the under sheet leaving enough free tubing to permit some movement of the child.

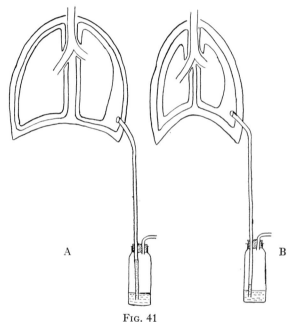

FIG. 41

Underwater seal drainage. (A) Inspiration—note rise of water in glass tube. (B) Expiration—note decreased capacity of chest and fall in the level of water in the glass tube.

Strong artery forceps should be available to clamp the tubing immediately should any emergency occur. Measurement of the drainage may be necessary at a given time each day if blood or pus is present. The tube should then be clamped (two clamps are a wise precaution), and the fluid measured. A fresh sterile bottle should then be used with the amount of fluid it contains marked on it.

Facts which must be understood by all members of the staff, including the domestic staff:

There must be no possibility of any part of the apparatus becoming disconnected. Should this occur, air would immediately rush into the pleural cavity and the lung would collapse.

The bottle should be maintained in a position at least 80-100 cm., 32 to 40 inches, below the level of the chest; if it is raised higher, with vigorous inspiratory effort, the fluid could be sucked into the pleural cavity; should it be lifted above the level of the chest, syphonage of fluid would occur into the pleural cavity.

REMOVAL OF THE CATHETER. Oscillations may cease when the lung is fully expanded, or the tube has become blocked with blood or pus. Clinical findings and X-ray will prove if it is the former, and usually on full expansion of the lung, the tube is removed. Whenever oscillations cease, the fact should be reported to the doctor in charge. A blocked drainage tube is of no value to the patient and could be harmful. Requirements depend on the method to be used. The stitch may be cut and the catheter quickly removed, applying immediately an airtight dressing. Alternatively, a purse string suture may be used if no dressing is desired.

REQUIREMENTS:

Equipment 1-5 *sterile*
1. 1 pr. stitch scissors.
2. 1 pr. dissecting forceps.
3. Gallipot for skin cleansing lotion.
4. Swabs.
5. Sealing dressing such as four layer postage stamp size of tulle gras.
6. Waterproof adhesive tape.

Extra sterile requirements for purse string suture:
1. Fine half circle cutting needle.
2. Needle holder.
3. Black silk No. 000.

AFTER CARE OF THE CHILD is concerned with the observation of respiration and ensuring that there is full expansion of both lungs. These children require very gentle handling and any indication of respiratory difficulty must be reported immediately.

BIBLIOGRAPHY

Aberdeen, E. (1965). Mechanical Pulmonary Ventilation in Infants. *Proc. R. Soc. Med*, **58**, 11.

Aestrup, P., Jorgensen, K., Anderson, O. S. & Engel, K. (1960). *Lancet*, **1**, 1035.

Ellison Nash, D. F. (1965). *Principle and Practice of Surgical Nursing.* 3rd ed. London: Arnold.

Flitter, H. H. (1962). *An Introduction to Physics in Nursing*, 4th ed., Unit 5. St. Louis: Mosby.

Harmer, B. & Henderson, V. (1955). *Principles and Practice in Nursing*, 5th ed., chap. 27. New York: Macmillan.

Jackson Rees, G. & Owen-Thomas, J. B. (1966). A technique of pulmonary ventilation with naso-tracheal tube. *Br. J. Anaesth.*, **38**, 901.

Lambert, V. (1968). Modern application of tracheostomy. *Nurs. Mirror*, **126**, 13.

Lancet (1962). Oxygen Therapy. **2**, 1093.

Ludman, H. (1967). Tracheostomy. *Nurs. Mirror*, **124**, 18.

McDonald, I. H. & Stocks, J. G. (1965). Prolonged naso-tracheal intubation. *Bri. J. Anaesth.*, **37**, 3.

Oppe, T. E. (1961). *Modern Textbook of Paediatrics for Nurses*, chap. 18. London: Heinemann.

Taverner, D. (1961). *Physiology for Nurses*, chap. 10. London: English Universities Press.

CHAPTER XIII

PROCEDURES RELATING TO THE
ALIMENTARY SYSTEM

Lubrication of oesophageal and gastric tubes; oesophagoscopy; gastric aspiration; gastric lavage; artificial feeding; gastric analysis; rectal lavage; colonic lavage; rectal examination.

LUBRICATION OF OESOPHAGEAL AND GASTRIC TUBES

IT will be noted that throughout the text, we have merely moistened the tubes to be passed either orally or by the nasal route.

THERE ARE SEVERAL REASONS FOR THIS:

1. It has been said by an older child, who was having a tube passed at intervals, that when the tube was warm and moist, it was easier to go down and there was no 'nasty' taste.

2. Lubricants such as liquid paraffin may well have a considerable aperient action, if the tube has to be passed at frequent intervals.

3. If specimens are being obtained for laboratory investigations, the use of lubricants may well alter the specimens.

4. There are considerable dangers associated with liquid paraffin being inhaled and causing lipoid pneumonia. Also, for the older child, the taste is unpleasant.

5. The use of glycerine and borax is also contra-indicated if used repeatedly, because of the marked toxic effect of borax.

A lubricant may be requested on occasion. Water soluble varieties such as KY jelly have no known harmful effects.

OESOPHAGOSCOPY

This is a direct vision examination of the oesophagus. It may be carried out:

1. In an effort to recover a foreign body which has become lodged in the oesophagus.

2. As an aid to diagnosis, or to determine progress in the presence of dysphagia, or suspected disease of the oesophagus.

3. To dilate the oesophagus when there is a stenosis.

PREPARATION FOR THE PROCEDURE. Oesophagoscopes of varying sizes will be required. These contain light carriers and sterilisation of the light carriers and flex can be carried out by immersion in biniodide of mercury 1:5000 for fifteen minutes. Alternatively, a formalin cabinet may be used. A powerful suction apparatus with adequate length of tubing from the suction bottle is essential. If the bottle contains approximately two inches of water it facilitates cleaning. Instruments and batteries must be tested and in working order. A bowl of sterile water is placed near the suckers for rinsing purposes.

REQUIREMENTS:

Trolley with sterile equipment on upper shelf:
1. Laryngoscope and three blades.
2. Oesophagoscopes (sizes as required).
3. Light carriers to fit, with bulbs.
4. 2 crocodile forceps.
5. Foreign body and biopsy forceps.
6. 3 to 4 suckers.
7. Oesophageal bougies (if required).
8. Swabs.
9. Stainless steel measuring tape.

Trolley—lower shelf:
1. 1 battery box and leads.
2. Receptacle for used swabs.
3. Receptacle for instruments.

In Addition:
Equipment for the administration of an anaesthetic.
Resuscitation equipment (Chapter XX).

PREPARATION OF THE CHILD. This procedure is done under anaesthesia and the child is prepared accordingly. The child is dressed in a cotton jacket with front opening. Premedication is given prior to the procedure, the drug, dose and time being in accordance with the instructions of the anaesthetist.

Correct positioning of the child on the theatre table is important. The head is extended so that the oesophagus is in a straight line.

AFTER CARE. There may be some degree of dysphagia afterwards and, if present, fluids are given in small quantities more frequently. Small, frequent milk drinks will help to alleviate pain if there is an oesophagitis. It is also preferable to have the child propped up as soon as possible to prevent reflux of gastric juices up the oesophagus. These would cause considerable irritation and pain.

If there has been difficulty in removing a foreign body, resulting in injury to the mucosa of the oesophagus, sterile fluids are given and an antibiotic may be ordered.

GASTRIC ASPIRATION

Gastric aspiration is performed to relieve the stomach and small bowel of gaseous distension and fluid content. It may be ordered in a variety of circumstances, as for example:

1. Mechanical obstruction such as intussusception, volvulus or atresia of a section of the alimentary tract.
2. Paralytic ileus.
3. Pre-operative preparation prior to surgery of the alimentary tract.

The danger of an ill infant with any form of intestinal obstruction inhaling regurgitated stomach content is very real. In these circumstances there should be no delay in passing a gastric tube to empty the stomach and, by leaving the tube in position and unclamped, allow free drainage of fluid or gas.

Paralytic ileus or paralysis of the intestinal muscles is associated with various conditions. It provides as effective an obstruction to the onward passage of bowel content as the mechanical type. A paralytic ileus may develop following an accident when the patient is suffering from shock. It is important to remember that in this instance solid food taken shortly before the accident will remain in the stomach for a much longer period and will not be removed by gastric aspiration. In such circumstances, gastric lavage would be required using a large gastric tube; thereafter a fine gastric tube may be introduced and left in situ.

The type of tube used is a matter of choice. A Ryle's tube with a weighted tip may be used, or an oesophageal tube which has larger holes may be considered wiser. The size used must not be larger than that which can be passed comfortably via the nose, as the tube may have to remain in position for a period of days.

PREPARATION OF THE CHILD.

This consists of explanation to the older child. The younger

child will require to have his arms splinted until he is used to the
tube and is no longer likely to pull it out.

REQUIREMENTS:

1. Ryle's or oesophageal tube 9-12 F.G., 4-6 E.G.
2. Cotton wool balls and paper tissues.
3. Gallipot with warm water.
4. 20 ml. syringe.
5. Litmus paper.
6. Water repellent sheet.
7. Receptacle for aspirate.
8. Receptacle for used swabs.
9. Vomit bowl and disposable towel.
10. Adhesive tape and scissors.
11. Restraining sleeves (Fig. 42).

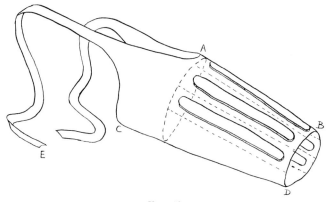

FIG. 42
The restrainer sleeve (see Appendix B for Measurements.)

METHOD. Two nurses are required; one to perform the procedure and the other to hold and comfort the child. Both should
wash and dry their hands. The child should be lying comfortably
in bed with one or more pillows. The nostrils are cleaned with
moist cotton wool. The tube is measured from the nape of the
nose to the tip of the xiphisternum. It is moistened and passed
approximately one to three inches beyond the measured point,
or until the aspirated material flows freely. Details of passing a

tube nasally are given under naso-gastric feeding. The aspirated material is tested with litmus paper; an acid reaction gives proof that the contents are from the stomach. The tube is then fixed to the cheek with adhesive tape. Aspiration with the 20 ml. syringe continues until the stomach is empty. It may be that on aspirating, only air is obtained; *the reason can be twofold:*

(*a*) the tube has curled up in the naso-pharynx and has not entered the stomach. The back of the throat should be examined, and the tube repassed if necessary.

(*b*) gas is being withdrawn from the stomach. Aspiration should be continued until the piston fails to be withdrawn and all the gas has been removed.

The tube is then left open and allowed to drain. This enables gas to be expelled and thus relieves distension.

Suction may be applied to the end of the tube and this can be obtained by using a 'three bottle method', or by the use of an

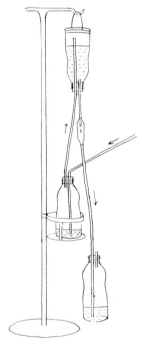

Fig. 43
Gastric suction by gravity
method.

electric pump. There are many types of pump on the market. The important factor in their use is that the suction must not be too strong. Should the eye of the tube be against the wall of the stomach, the mucosa may well be sucked into it and injured. Some machines have a mechanical cut-out device to avoid this and suction is, therefore, intermittent. The vacuum should be 12 cm. Hg or 5 in. Hg.

The 'three bottle system' is not as complicated as it might appear and is most effective. There is no need for clamps on the apparatus except when changing the bottles (Fig. 43).

GASTRIC LAVAGE

The stomach is washed out for the following reasons:

1. In cases of poisoning, in an effort to remove and dilute the poison.

2. Where there is irritation of the gastric mucosa due to causes other than poisoning; e.g., (a) gastro-enteritis, (b) mucus swallowed during the process of birth, and (c) in the infant with an upper respiratory tract infection due to the swallowing of infected material.

3. To cleanse and empty the stomach prior to specific operation on the stomach, or upper part of the alimentary canal. A gastric lavage may also be necessary for this reason prior to an emergency operation to ensure that the stomach is empty.

4. For diagnostic purposes. To assess the amount of residue as in a pyloric stenosis, or to obtain gastric washings.

This procedure requires sterilised equipment for an infant. For the older child, the equipment is clean and is always sterilised after use.

REQUIREMENTS:

1. Paper tissues.
2. Gallipot of warm sterile water for moistening the tube.
3. Oesophageal catheters, sizes according to age. For small infants—No. 15 F.G. or No. 8 E.G. For the older child—No. 20-24 F.G. or No. 12-14 E.G. Nutrient funnel is used for infants and a conical funnel for older children. Tubing 12 to 24 in. in length and a connecting tube.
4. Jug containing the required lotion, temperature 37·2°C or 99°F, placed in a bowl of warm water.

5. Lotion thermometer.
6. Water repellent sheet.
7. Floor mackintosh, basin or pail for return flow.
8. Measure for residue.
9. Vomit bowl and towel for the older child.
10. Receptacle for disposable items.
11. Receptacle for salvage.

Split pressure tubing 1 in. length available to slip on to oeso-phageal tube to place between the teeth if the older child should persist in biting the tubing. This is frequently necessary and has

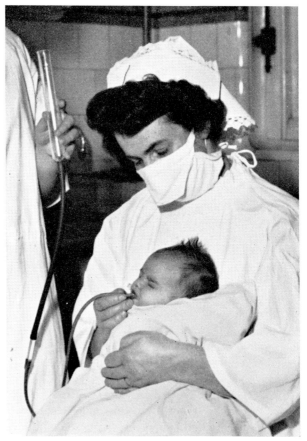

Fig. 44
Position of infant for gastric lavage

been found by the authors to save the use of a mouth gag which is a dangerous object with a struggling child.

Lotion to be used is dependent on the reason for the lavage. Certain poisons require specific antidotes; otherwise, normal saline is frequently ordered.

PREPARATION. Two nurses should always carry out this procedure and each must be aware of the dangers which might present themselves.

The child, if old enough, should have an explanation of what is about to happen. The position and correct restraining is of the utmost importance. It is preferable and considerably safer for the infant to be sitting upright on a nurse's knee, facing the operator, as in Figure 44.

The older child, if unable to be adequately held this way, may have to be in the semi-recumbent position in bed, positioned slightly on one side. The arms and legs must be well wrapped and tucked firmly away.

Important points to understand when carrying out a gastric lavage:

1. When passing the catheter should coughing occur, or any sign of respiratory distress, or cyanosis, the catheter must be withdrawn immediately.

2. Should there be any difficulty in passing the catheter, force should never be used. The fact must be reported. A fibrous narrowing of the oesphagus may exist and trauma could be caused.

3. The catheter may curl up at the back of the throat. To ensure that this does not occur, it is advisable to open the child's mouth gently and inspect the back of the throat.

4. The capacity of an infant's stomach may be as little as two ounces. Therefore, great care must be taken not to run in more fluid at one time than the stomach can safely hold (p. 194).

5. A nutrient funnel should be used for infants, as the narrow bore of the end reduces the rate of flow and the small capacity of the funnel (60 ml.) prevents overdistension of the stomach.

6. Regurgitation of fluid may easily lead to aspiration into the lungs. This is more likely with a weakly infant, or unconscious patient. Should regurgitation of fluid occur, invert the patient, lower the funnel and syphon back the fluid quickly. The catheter is removed and the airway cleared by using suction.

METHOD. Both nurses wash and dry hands. The assistant positions the child correctly and gives him as much comfort as possible during this very unpleasant procedure. The operating nurse assembles the apparatus, checks the temperature of the fluid, and measures the oesophageal tube. A useful guide is to measure from the nape of the nose to the tip of the xiphisternum, the latter being regarded as the lower end of the oesophagus. The catheter is held in one hand approximately one inch or more beyond the measured point. With the other hand, the tip is moistened and while the assistant holds the child's head, the catheter

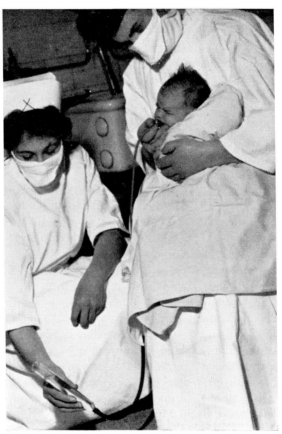

FIG. 45
Position of infant for the return of fluid during a gastric lavage.

is passed gently over the back of the tongue down the oesophagus into the stomach. If the child is old enough ask him to swallow just as the catheter goes over, this will make the passage easier. The catheter should not be forced or passed too quickly. Once the catheter is in position, it must be maintained and not allowed to slip through the fingers either one way or the other. The funnel is lowered to collect the residue which is emptied into a separate container. The obtaining of residue is proof of the correct position of the catheter.

If there is any difficulty, turn the child from one side to the other and if possible get him to cough. Not more than 15 ml. sterile water should be introduced until definite gastric residue has been obtained, then the lavage can proceed. The height of the funnel and the capacity will influence the force and the rate of flow, remembering the capacity of the child's stomach. Great care must be taken not to overfill the stomach and to ensure that all fluid given is syphoned back each time. The funnel is normally held six to twelve inches above the child's head. When the funnel is lowered to collect the return, it is kept upright (Fig. 45) until the equivalent amount of fluid has been obtained; it is then inverted into the bucket. This is necessary to ensure that fluid is not being retained. The lavage is continued until the return fluid is clear, or until the ordered amount of fluid has been used. For small infants this is only one pint of fluid. The return flow and residue is kept for inspection and, if necessary, analysis.

After the procedure the child should be comforted and returned to bed.

ARTIFICIAL FEEDING

There are various methods of feeding by artificial means. The method of choice depends upon various factors, and consideration of these must be made before the decision is taken as to which method will be employed.

1. Oesophageal and Gastric Gavage

The giving of a feed into the lower end of the oesophagus or stomach by passing a tube through the mouth. The tube is withdrawn on completion of the feed.

This method is used when it is considered unwise to leave a fine oesphageal tube in position, or when regular artificial feeding is not necessary. It is useful when nursing infants with the following conditions: prematurity, exhaustion in infants due to congenital heart disease accompanied by heart failure, and in acute respiratory distress.

The passage of a tube repeatedly via the nose would lead to irritation and trauma. It is never carried out in premature infants because of this danger. The passage of the tube only as far as the lower end of the oesophagus is usually preferred because it can be repeated at regular intervals without causing vomiting or gastric irritation. It is particularly advisable in premature infants, as gastric feeding may cause distension due to air becoming trapped in the stomach. If gastric gavage were carried out at three- or four-hourly intervals over a long period of time, there would be a great danger of injuring the gastric mucosa by repeatedly hitting the same point on the greater curvature of the stomach.

2. Continuous or Intermittent Artificial Feeding by the Naso-gastric Route

This is the giving of a feed directly into the stomach through a fine tube passed via the nostril to the stomach, and left in position throughout the period during which artificial feeding is required.

This is the method usually preferred as it is least disturbing to the child. It is used for the debilitated infant or child, or where there has been extensive injury. A very fine oesophageal or polyvinyl tube is used, which causes no irritation, and may be left in position for a period of two to three weeks without changing. Rubber feeding tubes are not used, as they cause considerable irritation when left down for a long period. Feeds can be given very slowly and are, therefore, more readily tolerated. The debilitated older child may have artificial feeds given only during the night, the tube being clamped off by day, allowing him to take diet and more readily encourage the return of his appetite. It is also the method used for the unconscious child. In deep coma, the cardiac sphincter is relaxed and allows the contents of the stomach to return to the pharynx. This may lead to regurgitation and aspiration of feed and it is, therefore, essential to give only small quantities very slowly.

PREPARATION OF THE CHILD FOR ARTIFICIAL FEEDING. Explanation to the older child is essential. If the tube is to remain in position for a longer period than one feed, it is necessary to restrain the arms of the younger child. The younger child can be held on a nurse's knee, positioned and wrapped as for a gastric lavage. The older child is most comfortable in the semi-recumbent position, and the unconscious child in the right lateral position with the head of the bed raised 30°.

Oesophageal or Gastric Gavage

REQUIREMENTS. The equipment is sterile for infants and sterilised after use for the older children.

1. Swabs.
2. Gallipot with warm water.
3. Nutrient funnel or 20 ml. syringe.
4. Tubing, six inches to twelve inches in length.
5. Oesophageal tube and connection or polyvinyl tube.
6. Small measure of sterile water.
7. Jug or bottle with feed warmed—temperature 37·2°C or 99°F when given.
8. Food thermometer.
9. Water repellent sheet.
10. Receptacle for used apparatus.
11. Receptacle for disposable items.

Size of oesophageal tube for premature or small infants is No. 9 F.G. or No. 4 E.G. Infants to older children—No. 12-14 F.G. or No. 6-8 E.G.

METHOD. Two nurses are required, one to hold and comfort the child; the other to perform the procedure. Both wash and dry their hands. The child is protected with a water repellent sheet. The apparatus is assembled by the nurse, the temperature of the feed is checked, and the oesophageal tube is measured from the nape of the nose to the tip of the xiphisternum. This can be accepted as the distance to the lower end of the oesophagus. Thus, if an oesophageal feed is to be given, the tube will be passed this length; if a gastric feed is to be given, it will be necessary to pass it from one to three inches further, depending on the size of the child. After measuring the tube, the assistant carefully wraps the child up, tucking the arms well out of the way. The other nurse moistens the tube, and, with one hand holding the funnel and the measured point of the tube, the other slowly and steadily passes the catheter over the back of the tongue. Should there be any coughing or respiratory distress, the tube is immediately withdrawn and re-passed when the child has recovered. If the tube is to be passed into the stomach, by lowering the funnel, syphonage of the gastric residue will prove that it is correctly positioned. Violent coughing would result should the catheter not be in the stomach. This would necessitate inverting the patient immediately, and removing the tube.

Once the tube is positioned, it must be held carefully and the fluid given slowly. The rate is determined by the condition of the child and a guide for an infant is that it should take as long to give as the child would take if the fluid were being given orally.

The capacity of the stomach increases to accommodate food or fluid, but in the small infant this may be as little as one ounce. The following table is a guide as to the capacity of the stomach in the first year of life (after Griffith and Mitchell).

at birth	= 1·0-1·2 oz.	30- 36 ml.
1 week	= 1·3-1·5 oz.	39- 45 ml.
2 weeks	= 2·0-3·0 oz.	60- 90 ml.
1 month	= 2·5-3·0 oz.	75- 90 ml.
3 months	= 3·3-4·5 oz.	99-135 ml.
6 months	= 4·5-6·0 oz.	135-180 ml.
1 year	= 7·5-9·0 oz.	225-270 ml.

Once the feed is given, the tubing is firmly nipped and the tube removed. The child should not be laid flat immediately, but held in a sitting position and comforted before being returned to bed.

Intermittent Naso-gastric Feeding

REQUIREMENTS:

Sterile equipment :

1. Swabs and cotton wool balls.
2. Gallipot with warm sterile water.
3. Nutrient funnel or 20 ml. syringe.
4. Six-inch length of rubber tubing.
5. Connection.
6. Naso-gastric feeding tube with spigot size 9 F.G. or 4 E.G. or polyvinyl tube.
7. Container with warmed feed—temperature 37·2°C, or 99°F when given.

Additional equipment :

   8. Lotion thermometer.
   9. Paper tissues.
  10. Litmus paper.
  11. Adhesive tape and scissors.
  12. Receptacle for used apparatus.
  13. Receptacle for disposable items.

METHOD. Where possible the infant or child is prepared and positioned as for a gastric lavage. If the child is unable to be moved from his cot, raising the top of the cot by 30° will lessen the risk of aspiration. The tube is measured in the same way and moistened. It is much finer and, as it has to stay in position for a period of time, it is passed by the nasal route. The nostril is cleansed if necessary with moist cotton wool and the tube is passed very gently up and over to the measured point. Force should never be used and the other nostril should be used if there appears to be any obstruction. The finer tube is more likely to enter the bronchus of a very ill or unconscious child without evidence of coughing. It is, therefore, essential that the gastric content be aspirated. Proof of the nature of the aspirate can be obtained by testing it with litmus paper, gastric juice being acid. When the tube is correctly positioned, it is strapped on to the cheek.

The feed is given either by attaching the funnel and tubing, or by using a syringe. With the latter method it is essential not to use force. The fine tube ensures that the feed is not given too quickly, but if force is used to give it, the jet impinges on the same spot on the stomach wall and over a period of time this could lead to ulceration. After the feed has been given, the tube is rinsed through by injecting a small quantity of water. A plastic spigot is then inserted. When a polyvinyl tube is used, a plastic clamp is applied to seal off the tube. If the patient is a small infant it is helpful to fit a tube-gauze cap on the infant's head and keep the tube in place underneath it. This will enable the infant to move his head without danger of pulling the tube out. The hands can be enclosed in mittens but it is important to check frequently to ensure that the infant's fingers are *not* constricted.

The tube which is in situ should be aspirated each time prior to feeding to ensure it is in the correct position. 5 ml. of water may be injected to find out if the tube is blocked. If it is blocked, and the blockage cannot be easily removed, then a new tube has to be inserted. Care must be taken not to give more than 5 ml. of water to a young infant, so that the total intake is not increased excessively. The time to be taken to give each feed depends on the individual requirements viz. the amount to be given, the size of the child, the condition of the child and the position in which he is to be nursed. After the feed is completed, if the child has to be moved, he should be moved gently, but if he is very ill, it is wise not to disturb him for at least half an hour after the feed has been given.

Continuous Artificial Feeding by Naso-gastric Route

This can be employed as has been suggested, during the night, being discontinued during the day to allow the child to take diet, or used to give feeds more slowly throughout the twenty-four hours.

REQUIREMENTS:

Sterile equipment for small infants:
1. Swabs and cotton wool balls.
2. Gallipot with warm water.
3. Flask with feed—temperature 37·2°C or 99°F.
4. Disposable intravenous giving set, or similar apparatus.
5. For infants and small children, a 60 ml. nutrient funnel and a twelve-inch and three-inch length of tubing.
6. Screw clip or plastic clamp.
7. 10 ml. syringe.

Additional equipment:
8. Lotion thermometer.
9. Hanger for flask and label.
10. Adhesive tape.
11. Litmus paper.
12. Receptacle for apparatus.
13. Receptacle for disposable items.
14. Infusion stand.

METHOD. The fine oesophageal feeding tube is passed as for intermittent feeding, and the gastric aspirant is tested. The intravenous set is connected to the flask and the air expelled from the tubing. It is connected to the patient's tube and allowed to drip slowly in, the rate of flow being adjusted as ordered.

For the young child, or unconscious patient, there would be a tremendous danger of aspiration of feed should the infusion begin to run suddenly more quickly. This method must, therefore, never be used for them without some modification. No more than the amount of feed equivalent to the capacity of the stomach should be in the reservoir. If an open nutrient funnel is being used, it should be approximately twelve inches above the child's head. The clip must be between the funnel and the drip connection. A swab should be placed on top of the open funnel and the whole apparatus removed, washed, and re-sterilised after the feed has been given.

The disposable type of giving set for paediatric use, which permits small quantities of fluid to be run into the reservoir, overcomes the danger of too much fluid being given in a short period.

Gastrostomy Feed

A gastrostomy is an opening into the stomach through the abdominal wall into which a catheter is passed. This form of artificial feeding is performed when there is some obstruction due to a stricture, or atresia, of the oesophagus. The catheter is kept in position and changed as is necessary every few weeks.

At operation, the skin is invaginated as in an unspillable inkpot to prevent regurgitation of gastric content around the tube.

The tube is only inserted two or three inches, depending on the size of the child and must be firmly secured. Most surgeons prefer a catheter of some plastic material, which is non-irritant. A self-retaining catheter may be inserted, though more normally, a Jacques type, which does not require the use of an introducer, is used.

REQUIREMENTS:

Sterile equipment :
1. Nutrient funnel.
2. Twelve-inch length of tubing.
3. Graded connection.
4. Container with warmed feed—temperature 37·2°C or 99°F.
5. Food thermometer.

6. Two ounces (60 ml.) sterile water.

7. Towel.

METHOD. An explanation is necessary for the older child who, when well enough, can participate with his own feeding. The child is made comfortable in usually the semi-recumbent position in bed, or up in a chair if well enough. The nurse washes and dries her hands, assembles the apparatus, and then checks the temperature of the feed. A towel is laid under the gastrostomy tube, the spigot is removed, and the connection attached. A small quantity of water is run into the tube and then the feed is given. The funnel should be kept just about the level of the

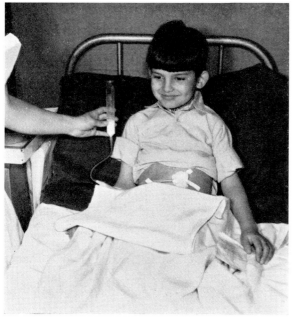

FIG. 46
Gastrostomy feed

abdomen and the feed allowed to run in slowly (Fig. 46). If the child is distressed, or retching, the feed will come up the funnel, and for this reason the funnel should always be only half filled, and once the child has recovered, the feed can be allowed to run in again slowly. After the feed has been given, the tube is cleaned with a small quantity of water and the spigot is replaced.

It is preferable not to lay the child down immediately after a gastrostomy feed and the child should be moved very gently.

The appearance of bile at the connection immediately the apparatus is assembled before the feed is given, should make the nurse suspect that the gastrostomy tube has passed through the pylorus into the duodenum. The matter should be reported and the tube may then be withdrawn slightly, or removed and re-passed.

Strict attention to oral hygiene is essential for any child having artificial feeds. It should be carried out routinely at feeding times. A child with a gastrostomy may be permitted to suck something pleasantly tasting during feeding. This is thought not only to give satisfaction, but also to stimulate the gastric juices.

The dressing around the gastrostomy tube is changed as is necessary. It is considered as a surgical dressing, and not part of the feeding regime.

GASTRIC ANALYSIS
(Augmented Histamine Test)

The gastric mucosa secretes gastric juice throughout the twenty-four hours, the amount varying with the age of the child. The rate of secretion is not constant, nor is the level of acidity. In the normal newborn infant, gastric acidity is relatively high but falls rapidly in the first ten days and then rises gradually to adult levels at 12 years.

Average normal gastric juice contains a high concentration of hydrochloric acid, organic material including mucin, enzymes, and inorganic constituents such as sodium, potassium, magnesium, chlorides and other salts. It also contains the important intrinsic factors required for the absorption of vitamin B.12.

Tests are performed to determine the presence of hydrochloric acid and the degree of acidity of stomach contents. There are different types of tests, but the one most frequently used at the present time is the Augmented Histamine Test. When gastric and duodenal ulcers are suspected, these can be readily confirmed by straight radiographs or fluoroscopy.

QUIREMENTS:

1. Flask marked 'fasting juice'.
2. Labelled specimen flasks (4).
3. 20 ml. syringe.

  4. Ryle's tube and spigot.
  5. Gallipot of warm water.
  6. Flask of normal saline—temperature 37·2°C or 99°F.
  7. Lotion thermometer.
  8. Swabs.
  9. 2 × 2 ml. syringes and needles No. 1 and 17.

Additional equipment :

  10. Vomit bowl and disposable towel.
  11. Adhesive tape and safety pin.
  12. Litmus paper.
  13. Suction apparatus.
  14. Histamine Acid Phosphate (increases gastric secretion).
  15. Anthisan (anti-histamine).
  16. Receptacle for apparatus and instruments.
  17. Receptacle for disposable items.

METHOD. The older child is given a simple explanation. He may be given books to read or toys to play with in an effort to distract him. Some attempt should be made to prevent the tantalising sight of the breakfast trolley.

Younger children should have their arms splinted. The test is performed after twelve hours fasting. In selected cases premedication may be prescribed.

Two nurses will be required and both should wash and dry their hands. One will hold the child in a comfortable position, either in bed, or on her knee, until the tube is passed. The second nurse cleanses the child's nostrils, then moistens the tube, and passes it as for a naso-gastric tube. The position of the tip of the catheter is checked radiologically; it should be at the greater curvature. Throughout the procedure, the child is kept lying on the left side in a semi-upright position.

The fasting juice is aspirated, measured, and put into the flask marked for that purpose. The stomach is washed out with normal saline, using a 20 ml. syringe, until the fluid returned is clear.

Minute 0: 'Basal juice' is aspirated using the pump at a 'sucking' pressure of 10-15 cm. of water.

Minute 40: An *intramuscular* injection of 'Anthisan' is given, dose according to doctor's written instruction.

Minute 60: (a) 'Basal' collection is discontinued. It is measured and kept.

(b) The child is given a *subcutaneous* injection of Histamine Acid Phosphate 0·04 mg./Kg. according to doctor's written instruction.

(c) The first collection of specimen 'A' is obtained.

Minute 80: Collection of specimen 'B' is started.

Minute 100: Collection of specimen 'C' is started.

Minute 120: Collection is completed.

All the specimens are put into the appropriately labelled flasks, which are then taken to the biochemical laboratory.

At the end of the collection, the catheter is removed. A mouth wash may be given to the older child followed by a light meal, and the infant is given a feed.

Throughout the procedure it is important to watch the child carefully for any signs of reaction. Medical aid should be summoned should any signs of flushing, faintness or headache be present.

Histamine Test

This is another method which is often used. The preparation and care of the child are the same as in the previous one.

REQUIREMENTS: These are the same as in the Augmented Histamine Test, with the addition of six (6) test tubes labelled respectively 2-7 and Piriton (anti-histamine drug).

METHOD. The child fasts for six (6) hours prior to the test.

6.30 a.m. The child is given an *intramuscular* injection of Piriton, dose according to doctor's written instruction.

7.00 a.m. The tube is passed and all the gastric contents are aspirated and put into the flask marked 'Fasting juice'. A Histamine injection is given *subcutaneously*, dose according to doctor's instruction.

7.15 a.m. and at subsequent ¼ hourly intervals, gastric contents are aspirated and placed in the appropriate test tubes.

8.30 a.m. Final specimen is obtained and the test is completed.

At the end of the collection, the catheter is removed. A mouth wash may be given to the older child followed by a light meal, and the infant is given a feed.

Throughout the procedure it is important to watch the child carefully for any signs of reaction. Should any signs of flushing, faintness or headache occur, the doctor is notified as soon as possible.

RECTAL LAVAGE

REASON. To cleanse the rectum of faeces. It may be ordered prior to surgery on the lower bowel, or examination of the rectum. It is not used as a treatment for constipation as such.

PRINCIPLES INVOLVED.

1. Use of an isotonic solution in the maintenance of a correct water and electrolyte balance.

An isotonic solution is one which has the same osmotic pressure as some other solution with which it is compared; e.g., the concentration of salts in the blood serum is 0·9 per cent and a solution of sodium chloride of the same concentration is termed an isotonic solution. Therefore, a solution of normal saline can be safely used without fear of causing any fluid or electrolyte imbalance.

In an abnormally dilated colon, such as occurs in Hirschsprung's disease, there is a greater surface area than normal. If a soap and water enema, made with tap water, is given, severe shock may arise from 'water intoxication'. This is due to the rapid diffusion of water into the circulation from the dilated bowel. Water intoxication is characterised by listlessness, apathy, fatigue leading to mental confusion, convulsions and coma.

2. Speed of insertion of fluid. It should be understood that the greater the height of the column of liquid the greater the pressure and the more rapid the dilation of the bowel; also the larger the catheter the more rapid the flow; similarly, the greater the drop when the funnel is lowered below the level of the anus, the greater will be the suction, and the more rapid the return. It is essential that the flow and return should be gentle and regular to avoid possible damage to the mucosa of the bowel and considerable discomfort to the patient. For an infant, the funnel is held approximately ten inches above the buttocks.

3. Temperature of fluid. It is advisable to do nothing which would alter the body temperature and the fluid when it is run in should be 37·2°C or 99°F. Too hot a temperature would injure the mucous membrane and too cold could produce shock.

PREPARATION AND CARE OF THE CHILD. A simple explanation is necessary, giving assurance that what is about to happen is not painful but may be uncomfortable. The child is turned on to the lateral position and kept warm and covered. A water repellent sheet is placed under the buttocks. Two nurses are required, one to hold the child and distract his attention with a story or running commentary about something else. A relaxed child is important. Discomfort will be much less likely and the whole procedure will be more easily carried out. It is absolutely essential that a child, who is to have this procedure repeated at regular intervals, should have the correct approach the first time. He will then accept it, and not be worried or upset by each subsequent time. If a child is distressed whether through fear or pain, the lavage should be discontinued and the fact reported.

REQUIREMENTS:

Large tray or trolley.
1. Two-pint or one-litre jug of warm normal saline, or other isotonic solution standing in a bowl of hot water.
2. Lotion thermometer.
3. Conical funnel, two feet length of tubing, connection and catheter No. 14 F.G. or No. 8 E.G. for an infant, up to No. 24 F.G. or No. 14 E.G. for a twelve-year-old.
4. Swabs.
5. Lubricant—KY jelly.
6. Water repellent sheet.
7. Receptacle for apparatus.
8. Receptacle for disposable items.
9. Bucket for return flow.

METHOD. The apparatus is assembled and the catheter lubricated. It is then inserted into the rectum for approximately two to four inches. The length of the infant's rectum is one and a half inches. At the age of twelve, it is approximately four inches. To note the presence of flatus invert the funnel below the level of water in a basin and bubbles, which may be quite explosive, will be seen if flatus is present. The catheter is then gently inserted further and gradually withdrawn until all flatus is passed. With the catheter in the original position and the tubing doubled to compress it and prevent any flow, the funnel is filled with fluid and lowered to expel any air. It is then raised to allow the fluid to flow gently in. Whenever the funnel is almost empty, it is lowered nearly to floor level to aid syphonage, but it is held upright to ensure the amount given has been returned. It is then inverted and the fluid emptied into a bucket. One or two pints ($\frac{1}{2}$-1 litre) may be given, depending upon the age and condition. The procedure must be discontinued if it causes distress. When the catheter is finally withdrawn, the funnel is lowered and the fluid is syphoned back as it is withdrawn. The return fluid is measured, its character noted, and the result reported. The equipment is cleaned and sterilised after use, and any disposable equipment is placed in a covered container.

AFTER CARE. Leave the child comfortable and happy. Should he desire to defaecate, give him the satisfaction of a bedpan, or, if possible, take him to the toilet, even though this may be considered unnecessary.

COLONIC LAVAGE

REASON.

1. Pre-operative preparation prior to surgery of colon or sigmoidoscopy.

2. Hirschsprung's disease.

PREPARATION AND CARE OF THE CHILD. As for rectal lavage.

REQUIREMENTS. As for rectal lavage, but a greater quantity of fluid is required.

METHOD. Commence as for rectal lavage, passing the catheter approximately eight inches to obtain flatus. A lavage is given, and when the fluid returned is clear, the child is turned on to his back, inserting the catheter a further four inches. The lavage is repeated until the fluid returned is clear. The child is then turned to the right lateral position and the process repeated until the fluid returned is clear. When the catheter is finally withdrawn, the funnel is kept low to allow syphonage of the return fluid as it is withdrawn. If the child is in any way distressed or in pain, discontinue the procedure and seek advice. An isotonic solution must be used. The amount depends on the child's needs, but normally two pints 1 (litre) are adequate.

When a lavage is being given to a child with Hirschsprung's disease, a greater amount of fluid may be required. This is dependent upon the severity of the child's condition and the reaction to the procedure should be decided by a trained nurse or doctor. It is unlikely that the fluid returned will become clear after the first few lavages, and this, therefore, cannot be the deciding factor. The lavage may have to be carried out daily, or twice daily for a period of more than one week.

RECTAL EXAMINATION

REASON. This examination is commonly a simple digital one which is carried out in the ward or outpatient department. It is an aid to diagnosis and is a routine procedure in a child with abdominal pain. A pelvic cellulitis and a pelvic abscess which has spread from an inflamed appendix can be felt. The presence of hard faeces can be noted.

REQUIREMENTS:

1. Container with finger cots or disposable gloves.
2. Paper tissues.
3. Petroleum jelly or KY jelly.
4. Receptacle for disposable items.
5. Water repellent sheet.
6. Napkin for infant.

METHOD. It is important to gain the child's co-operation by adequate explanations and reassurance. A relaxed child is much easier to examine. The older child is usually placed in the left lateral position, whereas the infant is placed in the dorsal position with the knees flexed. The water repellent sheet or napkin is placed under the buttocks. While the examination is carried out by the doctor, the nurse should hold the child's hands and keep the knees flexed.

BIBLIOGRAPHY

Brittain, J. D. (1966). *Practical Notes on Nursing Procedures*, 5th ed., chap. 15. Edinburgh: Livingstone.

Broom, B. (1961). Water intoxication. *Nurs. Times*, **57**, 1455.

Flitter, H. H. (1962). *An Introduction to Physics in Nursing*, 4th ed., pp. 109, 123. St. Louis: Mosby.

Fuerst, E. V. & Wolff, L. (1964). *Fundamentals of Nursing*, 3rd ed., Unit 14, Part 39. Philadelphia: Lippincott.

Harmer, B. & Henderson, V. (1955). *Principles and Practice of Nursing*, 5th ed., chap. 29. New York: Macmillan.

CHAPTER XIV

PROCEDURES RELATING TO THE URINARY SYSTEM

Collection of specimens of urine; catheterisation; bladder decompression; bladder irrigation; kidney function tests; renal biopsy; cystometrogram.

COLLECTION OF SPECIMEN OF URINE

EXAMINATION of urine is essential as an aid to diagnosis and as an assessment of progress in conditions affecting the urinary tract. These conditions include infections and diseases of the urinary tract; e.g., nephritis and nephrosis and metabolic disorders; i.e. diabetes mellitus, galactosaemia and phenylketonuria.

There are various methods of collecting a specimen of urine but in all cases it is important to send the specimen or collection of urine as soon as possible to the laboratory. It must be kept in a cool place until tested.

The passing of a catheter into the bladder solely for the purpose of obtaining a specimen of urine is generally not advisable, owing to the risk of infection. There are, however, occasions when this method must be adopted. The following methods have been found by the authors to be simple and reliable, proving adequate for the collection of urine for examination purposes and being less upsetting to the child.

Method for the Male Infant

A urine collecting bag can be used. The napkin area is carefully cleaned with soap and water and dried thoroughly. The bag is attached, ensuring that the penis is well placed in the opening of the bag. The adhesive covering should not be removed from the part which will be over the scrotum. The aperture may be enlarged to include the scrotum if leakage is occurring, but the adhesive must not become adherent to the scrotum.

Male Infant up to Six Months Old—Alternative Method

This method is not to be recommended if disposable bags are

available, as there is an element of risk using a test tube if suitable precautions are not taken.

REQUIREMENTS:

1. Three pieces of adhesive tape $\frac{1}{2}$ in. wide, 3 in. long.
2. Two pieces 2 in. long.
3. Test tube.

METHOD. The test tube is prepared by applying one 2 in. length of strapping round the edge of the rim. This is a safety precaution, to avoid injury should the rim of the test tube have any imperfections not detected by the naked eye. The 3 in. lengths are attached evenly longitudinally at the top of the test tube and the 2 in. piece is used to fix the ends (Fig. 47). The

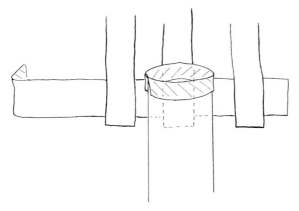

FIG. 47
Preparation of a test tube for collection of urine

napkin area is then carefully washed with soap and water, dried, and the test tube is applied (Fig. 48). Adhesive tape is not applied to the scrotum as this causes considerable pain when removed. The napkin is then applied, keeping the test tube visible. As soon as adequate urine has been obtained, the adhesive tape is gently removed using a swab with methylated ether. The urine is then transferred to a container which can be sealed; it is then labelled, stating the time the specimen has been obtained, and sent either to the laboratory or to the ward test room.

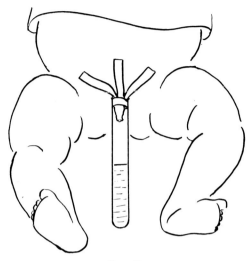

Fig. 48
Collection of a single specimen of urine from a
male infant.

Method for the Female Infant

A disposable urine collection bag is used.

REQUIREMENTS:

Sterile equipment :
1. Gallipots.
2. Swabs.
3. Container for urine.

Additional equipment :
4. Urine collecting bag.
5. Cleansing lotion.
6. Scissors.
7. Receptacle for disposable equipment.

METHOD. The nurse first washes and dries her hands, then she washes the infant's napkin area and dries it carefully. The hands are then washed and dried again. Using sterile swabs and cleansing lotion, the external genitalia is cleaned, working from above down either side of the labia until the area has been adequately

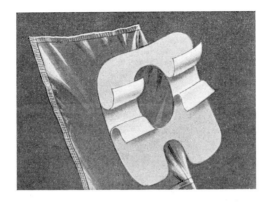

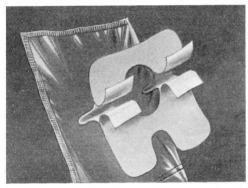

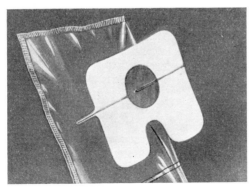

FIGS. 49, 50, 51

U-Bag. Demonstrates method of pleating to make
the aperture smaller. (Reprinted by kind permission
of C. F. Thackray Ltd.)

cleansed. The direction is important and is always from above downwards in an attempt to prevent the transfer of organisms from the perineum to the urethra and vagina. The area is dried carefully. The protective backing is then removed from the bag and it is applied from below working upwards. The adhesive is pressed carefully to the skin starting at the bridge of skin separating the rectum from the vagina, ensuring that the adhesive is firmly attached to the skin (Fig. 49). This type of bag has the advantage that the child need not be restrained, and indeed need not be confined to bed. The bag is a double container permitting no return flow thus avoiding leakage. The plastic spot at the

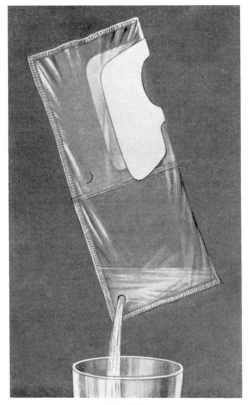

FIG. 52
Urine collecting bag. Demonstrates method of emptying during 24 hours collection of urine. (Reprinted by kind permission of C. F. Thackray Ltd.)

lower end of the bag is removed for emptying purposes and sealed with Sellotape. Figures 49-51 demonstrate the method of pleating to make the aperture smaller. The napkin can then be attached loosely, pinned at either side at the waist. As soon as an adequate amount of urine has been obtained, the bag is gently removed, using methylated ether. The urine is transferred to a suitable container, labelled, and sent to the laboratory or ward test room (Fig. 52).

Male or Female Infant—Alternative Method

A CLEAN CATCH SPECIMEN.

The napkin area is washed and dried carefully. The napkin is left open. The lid of the sterile container should be loosened but not taken off. The infant is fed and the urine caught in the container if voided during the feed.

For the Older Child—Mid-Stream Specimen of Urine

A sterile container for the specimen is required.

Whenever possible, this procedure should be performed when the child is up at the toilet. It should be explained exactly what is required of him.

METHOD. The child is asked to void urine into the toilet or urinal. After a small amount has been passed, the flow is directed into the sterile container for the specimen. The voiding is then completed. The specimen is labelled, and sent to the laboratory with the appropriate form.

24 hours Collection of Urine
Method for Male Infant

REQUIREMENTS:

1. 2 in. wide Paul's tubing, length adequate to reach the container for the urine at the end of the bed, and to allow the child to be moved for bedmaking and feeding.
2. Adhesive tape.
3. Scissors.
4. Restrainers for ankles.
5. Urine collection bag.

METHOD. After a bath, or cleansing of the napkin area, the

penis and scrotum are placed within the Paul's tubing, which is attached to the skin with adhesive tape.

The other end of the Paul's tubing is inserted into the collecting bag at the end of the bed. The napkin can be put on loosely and the ankles restrained. By placing the bag at the end of the bed, there is no risk of it being knocked by the cot sides, and it is less

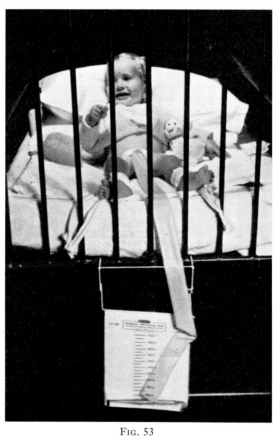

FIG. 53
Twenty-four hour collection of urine from male infant with Paul's tubing and disposable bag.

likely that the bedclothes will be tucked in over the Paul's tubing (Fig. 53). A $\frac{1}{2}$-hourly check should be made to ensure drainage is satisfactory.

This method is also most satisfactory for collecting urine over a long period. By inserting both the penis and the scrotum into the 2 in. Paul's tubing, leakage is prevented and the possibility of fixing adhesive tape tightly round the penis is avoided.

24 Hours Collection of Urine
Method for Male or Female Infant

A simple and satisfactory method of collecting urine over a long period is by using the Cambridge (Chiron) urine collection bag, complete with tubing which can be inserted into a collecting bag placed at the end of the bed. Application of the bag is as described on p. 208.

The plastic chair with potty (Fig. 54) is useful for obtaining a 24-hour collection of urine from an infant. Pillows are used to support the legs and to prevent dependent oedema.

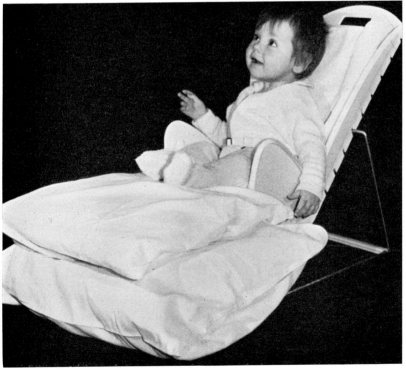

FIG. 54
Chair for infant with potty incorporated

CATHETERISATION

This is a procedure whereby the urinary bladder is emptied by artificial means.

It is undertaken for a variety of reasons :

1. AID TO DIAGNOSIS: (*a*) Diabetic coma.
   (*b*) Injury to bladder.
   (*c*) To ascertain the amount of urine remaining in the bladder after voiding.
   (*d*) Occasionally in urinary infection.

2. TO RELIEVE RETENTION OF URINE. This is only done as a last resort, when all other methods have failed.

3. PRE-OPERATIVE MEASURE. It is only undertaken when specifically ordered by the doctor, and again as a last resort if the child has failed to empty the bladder normally.

4. A CATHETER MAY BE PASSED AND LEFT IN POSITION: (*a*) to avoid contamination of dressings or exposed healing areas, (*b*) in an unconscious child to ensure adequate emptying of the bladder, and (*c*) to maintain an accurate fluid balance in metabolic disorders.

If the catheter is to be retained for any length of time, a self-retaining catheter is used. A Foley's catheter is ideal in such circumstances.

REQUIREMENTS:

Sterile equipment :
1. Swabs and cotton wool balls.
2. Gallipot with warmed cleansing lotion.
3. Gallipot for wrung out cotton wool balls.
4. 3 prs. forceps.
5. 2 catheters.
6. Receiver.
7. Container for specimen.
8. 3 dressing towels.
9. Sterile gloves (if desired).

Additional equipment :
10. KY jelly or sterile liquid paraffin if desired.
11. Receptacle for salvage.

12. Receptacle for instruments.
13. Receptacle for disposable items.
14. Label and form for specimen.
15. Book for child.
16. Good light; e.g., Anglepoise lamp.

It is essential to have the co-operation of the child while carrying out a catheterisation. A child who is frightened and restless will not be easily catheterised and this increases the danger of trauma, and the risk of contamination. It is not difficult to pass a catheter when a child is lying quietly; it is quite another matter if the child is tense or distraught.

The following method has been found by the authors to be one which can be carried out quickly and simply and causes the least upset to the child.

METHOD. Three nurses will be required, one to hold the child's legs in the correct position, the second to hold a book propped up on the child's chest to keep the instruments out of view and read to the child, and the third is the performer. The performer washes and dries her hands and with forceps wrings out about eight swabs, placing them in a gallipot. Using the same forceps, one catheter is moistened or lubricated if desired and placed in the receiver. The child is placed in position and a good light is directed at the vulval region.

Still using forceps, the performer cleanses the labia from above towards the perineum, cleansing each side and then the centre, using each swab only once and repeating as often as is necessary. These forceps are then discarded. The towels are placed in position, one covering each leg and joining over the abdomen, and the third is placed on the table between the legs up to the perineum. The receiver is now brought over on to the table or bed, and with the left hand the labia are separated. Only when the urinary meatus can be clearly seen lying above the vaginal orifice is the final cleansing performed, using the remaining pair of forceps. The catheter is then held with a gauze swab about two inches from the tip and is gently introduced (Fig. 55); alternatively a glove may be worn. The catheter is then held with the left hand while the container for the specimen is held with the right. The bladder is allowed to empty slowly, the catheter removed, and the labia dried. The child is then returned to bed after she has been comforted and given a reward.

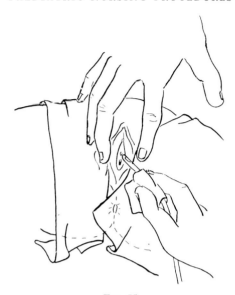

FIG. 55
Catheterisation of female child

The introduction of a catheter into the bladder is not undertaken unless absolutely necessary.

Foley's Self-retaining Catheter

Additional requirements for passing Foley's catheter :

Sterile water and 5 ml. syringe. When this type of catheter is introduced, the balloon is inflated with the appropriate amount of sterile water marked on the catheter and the bung is then firmly pushed into position. Vulval swabbing should be carried out 4-hourly when the catheter is left *in situ*. It is carried out in the same manner as cleansing prior to catheterisation and is important in the prevention of ascending infection to the bladder or kidneys.

Dangers of Catheterisation

1. Infection may easily spread through faulty technique. Organisms can be introduced into the bladder leading to an upward spread of infection.

2. Poor technique may cause trauma which in turn predisposes

to infection. This can be caused by the use of force in a tense child, or using too large a catheter.

Male patients are not catheterised by the nursing staff because of the danger of trauma. Greater skill and care are necessary on account of the presence of urethral valves and the angle of the urethra. The use of a lubricant such as KY jelly, or simply a moist catheter, is advocated by many for female and male catheterisation.

RETENTION OF URINE

Urine is excreted from the kidneys into the bladder where it is retained until the bladder is grossly distended.

Retention of urine may be caused by fear. This can be due to painful micturition, or merely strange surroundings; a bedpan, or fear of having an accident in bed. The latter three are all uncommon with children and are usually overcome with encouragement. The tap left running, additional fluid intake, and heat applied to the abdomen all help, but the important factor is a nurse, who can gain the child's confidence and help him to overcome his fear. When micturition is likely to be painful, if possible, the child should be given a hot bath and, if necessary, even allowed to void in the bath.

Retention may also be due to nerve damage, or temporary oedema causing pressure on the nerves in the bladder wall and sphincter, following an operation in the region of the bladder or lumbar spine, or when there has been spinal injury causing temporary or permanent paralysis. With such children it is essential to observe if they are voiding an adequate amount of urine at a time. It is not enough to note if the napkin or drawsheet is wet; the actual stream should be watched. Should the child dribble when crying or being moved, stress incontinence is present, the bladder being full and only the overflow voided. A distended bladder will soon lose tone should such a situation be allowed to persist for long.

BLADDER DECOMPRESSION

A grossly distended bladder should not be emptied rapidly because of the danger of damage to the bladder wall. This is especially liable to occur when the distension has been over a considerable time. Distension may occur where there is some urethral obstruction, such as urethral valves or bladder neck obstruction. Decompression can be carried out quite simply by clamping the catheter, releasing it every hour, and withdrawing 60 ml. urine.

DECOMPRESSION AND DRAINAGE by methods other than the use of a penile catheter may be necessary to ensure adequate clearance of residual urine from the bladder or from a grossly hydronephrotic kidney when the distension of the pelvis and calyces causes stasis of urine resulting in infection. In such instances, suprapubic cystostomy, nephrostomy, or ureterostomy has to be performed.

When a suprapubic drainage is required, an opening is made directly into the bladder through the abdominal wall and a self-retaining catheter is inserted. When a nephrostomy is performed, the catheter is inserted directly into the pelvis of the kidney.

A perineal urethrostomy is an opening made through the perineum into the urethra, through which a catheter is passed into the bladder. One reason for the bypassing of the penile urethra is to facilitate healing after plastic operations have been carried out, such as in a hypospadias deformity of the penis.

In all these types of drainage, sterile connection tubing and a collecting vessel, preferably a disposable plastic bag, and stand should be in readiness for the child's return from the theatre. Initially, restraining bands will be necessary, to ensure that the younger child, or the child recovering from anaesthesia, cannot pull out the tubing or catheter. Accurate measuring and charting of the fluid is essential. Daily cleaning and sterilisation of tubing as well as the collecting vessel, if these are not of the disposable type, is necessary to prevent ascending infections. To get rid of debris before sterilisation, the tubing should be run through with water from the tap, but preferably disposable tubing should be used.

Continuous Bladder Suction

This may be necessary to ensure a continually empty bladder following surgery of the bladder or urethra. An electric suction pump is used. The vacuum should not be high, 12 cm. Hg or 5 in. Hg.

BLADDER IRRIGATION

Bladder irrigation may be intermittent or continuous. With

a gravity apparatus, intermittent bladder irrigation is of use in cleansing the bladder of debris in long standing infections, or in an endeavour to remove a blood clot after operation. Catheterisation will be necessary if an indwelling catheter has not been already inserted.

Requirements and method for irrigation are the same whether a urethral or suprapubic catheter is used.

Intermittent Irrigation

REQUIREMENTS:

Sterile equipment :
1. Swabs and cotton wool balls.
2. Gallipot with cleansing lotion.
3. 2 prs. dissecting forceps.
4. Bladder syringe.
5. Jug for irrigation fluid, temperature 40·6°C or 105°F, e.g. normal saline, biniodide of mercury 1:1000, Acriflavine 1:1000.
6. Large receiver.
7. Water repellent sheet.
8. Lotion thermometer.

Additional equipment :
9. Receptacle for salvage.
10. Receptacle for instruments.
11. Receptacle for disposable items.

METHOD. Using forceps, the end of the catheter is cleansed and placed on the sterile sheet. The temperature of the lotion is tested and should be 100°F when given. The syringe is filled and not more than 30 ml. of the lotion is injected very slowly into the bladder. It is important to ensure that no air is injected as this causes pain and discomfort.

When ileal loop conduit or nephrostomy drainage is being irrigated, it must be remembered that each has a very limited capacity and not more than 15 ml. fluid should be instilled at a time unless otherwise ordered. This procedure should not be carried out if it causes pain. No force must be used to inject the fluid. The fluid must be measured and a return obtained before a further amount of fluid is injected.

Continuous or Intermittent Bladder Irrigation with a Gravity Apparatus

This may be ordered as a post-operative measure when there has been major surgery in the pelvic region, or in the treatment of long standing infection. It is considered less upsetting than repeated irrigation by syringe. The need for bladder irrigation has been considerably lessened since the introduction of anti-biotics. Long standing urinary infections are now much less prevalent.

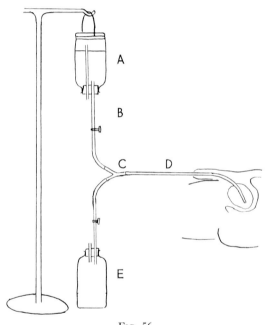

FIG. 56
Duke's apparatus for intermittent bladder irrigation

The apparatus is assembled and sterilised ready for use (Fig. 56):
1. Fill the reservoir A with measured fluid. Fix reservoir to stand and tighten clip on tube CE.
2. Lay tube CD on a sterile towel and clamp.
3. Release clamp CD and lift the tube to the height of the reservoir. Allow the fluid to run through and expel the air.

4. Lower tube CD and connect to the bladder and allow not more than 30 ml. fluid to run into the bladder. Close clip BC.

5. To empty the bladder open clip CE. This is left open until it is time to irrigate again.

Tidal Drainage

This means of drainage is rarely employed with children. It is used when it is thought desirable to encourage the natural filling and emptying of the bladder. The bladder is allowed to fill to an estimated amount and emptied by syphonage.

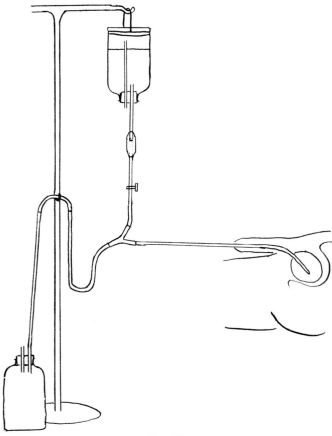

FIG. 57
Tidal drainage

The apparatus must be sterilised. Allow fluid to run through and expel air. It is allowed to run at 60 drops per minute and care must be taken to have the tubing only 2 in. above the symphysis pubis and 7 in. between '∩' tube and 'Y' tube, otherwise, damage could be done to the bladder by over-distension. When the bladder has become filled, the fluid rises in the system to the same level then flows over the '∩' tube down into the receptacle, thus emptying both the bladder and tubing by syphonage. The process restarts automatically. There must be no air in the catheter or tubing leading to it. The glass dripper must have an opening into it and the end of the outflow must not dip into the fluid of the receptacle. The tubing should be pressure tubing, i.e., of a large bore and thick walled. The lotion used is at room temperature and the choice of fluid is as for bladder irrigation (Fig. 57).

KIDNEY FUNCTION TESTS

Apart from chemical tests of the urine which the nurse can carry out in the ward, specific tests are done in the biochemical laboratory. These determine the efficiency of the kidneys.

The functions of the kidneys include excretion of waste products, the regulation of ionic balance, acid-base balance, and water balance of the body. These functions regulate the composition and volume of the blood plasma and also maintain and preserve osmotic pressure of the blood. In diseases affecting the kidneys, the functions of the kidneys may be altered or indeed may fail.

1. Urea Concentration Test

The test is used to determine the efficiency of the kidneys with regard to their urea excreting function. Urea is nitrogenous waste matter, one of the end-products of protein metabolism. For this test it is prepared in an artificial form.

PREPARATION OF THE CHILD. The child has nothing to eat or drink after his supper on the night previous to the test.

METHOD. 6 a.m. The child is asked to empty his bladder and the urine is put into a specimen glass.

15 grammes of urea are dissolved in 100 ml. of water and given to the child to drink.

He is asked to pass urine at 7 a.m., 8 a.m., 9 a.m. All the specimens are labelled and sent to the biochemical laboratory.

Three specimens of urine are necessary because the urea may
act as a diuretic, giving low readings of the first two specimens.
Low urea concentrations are obtained in nephritis or where
urinary outflow is blocked. In these cases, the blood urea is
raised.

2. Urea Clearance Test

This test involves a comparison between the percentage of urea
in the blood and in the urine. It demonstrates the efficiency of
the kidney to remove excess urea from the blood. A 24-hour
collection of urine is obtained. The time of commencement and
completion of the collection must be accurate and recorded on the
form, as an assessment is made on the average flow per minute.
The usual diet is given during the test. A specimen of blood is
obtained during the collection.

3. Concentration Test

This test measures the ability of the kidneys to concentrate
urine. Inadequate concentration of urine indicates some disorder
of the tubules of the kidneys.

PREPARATION OF THE CHILD. No fluids are given after 6 p.m.
on the day before the test.

METHOD. Any urine passed during the night is saved. At
6 a.m. the child is asked to empty his bladder—this urine is added
to any voided during the night. Three further specimens of
urine are obtained at intervals of one hour. All the specimens are
labelled, and sent with the necessary form to the biochemical
laboratory.

4. Creatinine Clearance Test

Creatinine is derived from the breakdown of muscle creatine
phosphate. The amount produced per day is relatively constant,
and is excreted by the kidneys. The normal range in the newborn
is 7-10 mg. per kg. per day, and in children 20-30 mg. per kg.
per day.

METHOD. Urine is collected for 24 hours. At the end of the
collection, a venepuncture is performed and 5 ml. of blood is

withdrawn, placed into a test tube and allowed to coagulate. The test is performed on the blood serum.

The collection of urine and the specimen of blood are labelled. These are sent, together with the necessary form containing the name, age, height and weight of the child, to the biochemical laboratory.

5. Addis Sediment Count

This test is carried out to determine any impairment in kidney function. Formed elements; i.e., red blood cells, white blood cells and casts, are normally found in small quantities in all urine specimens, provided intensive search is made for these elements. A sample of the urine is centrifuged and the sediment examined microscopically.

METHOD. No fluids are given after 4 p.m. All urine passed from 7 p.m. to 7 a.m. is collected, measured, and recorded.

CYSTOMETROGRAM

REASON. This test is an aid to diagnosis. It is used to determine the pressure within the bladder during voiding. Where there is an obstruction at the external sphincter, or at the outlet of the bladder, the pressure within a full bladder will be higher than normal and ureteric reflux may occur.

TECHNIQUE. The most accurate measurements are obtained when suprapubic percutaneous catheterisation is performed. Two intravenous cannulae (Intra-caths) are passed directly into the bladder; one is used to fill the bladder at a physiologically accepted rate (approximately 2 ml. per minute in an infant); the second catheter is used for recording purposes.

Alternatively, recordings can be taken after catheterisation per urethra and artificial filling of the bladder.

PREPARATION OF THE CHILD. An adequate explanation is given to the older child and his co-operation gained. Sedation will be advisable for the young child or infant. The procedure is not distressing once the initial puncture has been performed. It is however tedious, taking approximately two hours when a series of recordings are required.

It is desirable that the patient has a full bladder before starting the procedure. The child who is old enough is therefore encouraged to drink copiously one hour prior to the test and discouraged from voiding urine. Suitable books or toys should be provided, dependent upon the age of the child.

When suprapubic catheterisation is performed, a local anaesthetic is given unless the child has a lack of sensation below the waist; e.g., spina bifida, traumatic paraplegia.

REQUIREMENTS:

1. Swabs and cotton wool balls.
2. 2 gallipots.
3. 3 prs. dissecting forceps.
4. Receiver.
5. 2 catheters and spigot.
6. 2 medium intravenous cannulae (Intra-caths) when suprapubic puncture is performed.
7. 1 intravenous giving set.
8. 1 intravenous giving set with 100 ml. chamber.
9. 20 ml. syringe.

Additional equipment :

10. 1 flask sterile water.
11. 1 flask normal saline for filling bladder.
12. Cleansing lotion.
13. Container for specimen of urine.
14. Recording apparatus—electronic pressure transducer.
15. Label and form for specimen of urine.
16. Receptacle for salvage.
17. Receptacle for disposable items.
18. Receptacle for instruments.

AFTER CARE.

1. Haematuria if present is reported. This is usually slight and should not normally persist longer than twenty-four hours.

2. Leakage from the suprapubic puncture seldom occurs, but should be watched for.

3. Following the suprapubic method, catheterisation may be carried out to determine the amount of residual urine.

4. Suprapubic pressure to aid voiding in the paralysed child should be very gentle to avoid leakage from the suprapubic puncture.

P.N.P.—I

RENAL BIOPSY

REASON. This is a procedure which is an aid to diagnosis and which can often give an indication as to prognosis and response to treatment in children suffering from nephritis. Specimen of renal tissue is obtained and examined by electronic microscopy. PREPARATION OF THE CHILD. Before renal biopsy is carried out, treatment is given to reduce oedema and proteinuria. This may take 10 to 14 days, after which time an intravenous pyelogram is carried out to determine the efficiency of the kidneys. At the same time, a 'marker' is placed over the proposed site of puncture. The X-ray will show whether the 'marker' is placed in the correct position. Nurses must take care not to remove the 'marker'.

The following day, the child is prepared for the biopsy. This entails pre-operative preparation (see Chapter V). The procedure is carried out in the operating theatre.

CARE OF THE CHILD. Haemorrhage following biopsy is the principal danger. It is, therefore, important to handle the child carefully and special care should be taken when lifting the child from the trolley on to his bed.

On return from theatre, post-operative care is commenced with special emphasis on the following points:

1. The first urine voided is examined for blood. This is usually present for twenty-four hours after this procedure is carried out.

2. Pulse rate is recorded every hour for twelve hours, and two-hourly for twenty-four hours thereafter.

3. Blood pressure is checked four-hourly for twenty-four hours.

4. Any swelling or discolouration over the site should be watched for and reported. The wound is left without a dressing.

5. If the child has previously been allowed up, he is confined to bed for forty-eight hours following the biopsy.

BIBLIOGRAPHY

Flitter, H. H. (1962). *An Introduction to Physics in Nursing*, 4th ed., p. 108. St. Louis: Mosby.

Garb, S. & Sporne, P. (1962). *Nurse's Manual of Laboratory Tests*. London: Heinemann.

Harmer, B. & Henderson, V. (1955). *Principles and Practice of Nursing*. 5th ed. New York: Macmillan.

Hector, W. (1968). *Modern Nursing, Theory and Practice*, 4th ed., chap. 25. London: Heinemann.

Mason Brown, J. J. (1962). *Surgery of Childhood.* London: Arnold.
Murphy, J. J., Schoenberg, H. W. & Tristan, T. A. (1961). Analysis of neurogenic dysfunction of the lower urinary tract. *Br. J. Urol.,* **33,** 410.
Thomson, W. A. R. (1966). *Calling the Laboratory,* 2nd ed. Edinburgh: Livingstone.
Urine Testing. Uroscopy by Noughts and Crosses (1962). *Lancet,* **1,** leading article.
Wilson Nash, D. F. (1965). *Principles and Practice of Surgical Nursing,* 3rd ed., chap. 35. London: Arnold.

CHAPTER XV

PROCEDURES AND TREATMENT RELATING TO THE CARDIO-VASCULAR SYSTEM

Venepuncture; fontanelle tap; puncture of the jugular vein; puncture of the femoral vein; venesection; scalp vein infusion; blood transfusion; exchange transfusion; subcutaneous infusion; bone marrow puncture.

VENEPUNCTURE

REASONS. This procedure is carried out by the doctor. A vein is punctured for the following reasons:

A. To obtain a specimen of blood:
1. For biochemical investigation; e.g., estimation of blood urea.
2. For bacteriological investigation to culture bacteria.
3. To estimate the erythrocyte sedimentation rate.

B. To inject substances into the blood stream; e.g., iron, pentothal, glucose, saline, blood and opaque media.

REQUIREMENTS:

Sterile equipment :
1. Swabs.
2. Cleansing lotion in container.
3. Syringes; sizes according to the purpose required, e.g. 2 ml. for erythrocyte sedimentation rate: 5 ml. for culture.
4. Needles No. 12 or 14.
5. Appropriate container for specimen of blood.

If the specimen of blood is for bacteriological investigation the following additional sterile items will be required:
6. 2 cleansing lotions in containers.
7. Sterile towel.
8. Dissecting forceps.

Additional equipment :
9. Rubber tubing or tourniquet.
10. Water repellent sheet.

11. Citrate 3·8 per cent.
12. Receptacle for instruments.
13. Receptacle for disposable items.

PREPARATION OF THE CHILD. If the child is old enough the procedure should be explained to him. The child must be re-assured and the syringe should be kept out of his sight. It is often difficult to get into a child's vein so that the procedure may take longer than usual. The nurse places the water repellent sheet over a pillow and places the child's arm in the supine position, applying pressure over the area above the elbow joint. As soon as the doctor has withdrawn the needle, the nurse releases her grip, and applies a dressing and pressure over the puncture. If a drug or other substance is to be injected the nurse will release the pressure over the elbow area as soon as blood enters the syringe. When the injection is completed, pressure is applied over the punctured area until there is no oozing from the puncture. This prevents loss of the substance injected and also prevents the formation of a haematoma.

FONTANELLE TAP

This is a method of obtaining blood from an infant during the first year of life where the anterior fontanelle is still patent. A short thick needle is inserted into the posterior midline of the anterior fontanelle to reach the longitudinal sinus.

PREPARATION OF THE CHILD. Shaving of the head should only

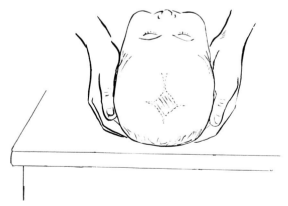

FIG. 58
Position of child for fontanelle tap

be done on instructions from the doctor. The infant is wrapped in a blanket and the crown of the head is held level with the edge of the table. Light flexion of the head may be necessary and any movement of the head prevented (Fig. 58).

As soon as the needle is withdrawn, the head is raised quickly and firm pressure is applied to the punctured point. The infant should not be returned to his cot until the nurse has reassured herself that no oozing of blood or serum is present.

REQUIREMENTS. The requirements are the same as for a venepuncture except that the needles are small and thick with a short bevel.

PUNCTURE OF THE JUGULAR VEIN

This is another method by which blood may be obtained from a small child. The position the child has to adopt will frighten him so reassurance will be necessary.

A pillow is placed on the edge of the table and the child's head placed on it, turned to the side, and well extended over the edge of the table. It is important that the child's head does not move during the procedure, but crying will distend the vein, facilitating entry into the vein (Fig. 59).

As soon as the doctor removes the needle, pressure must be

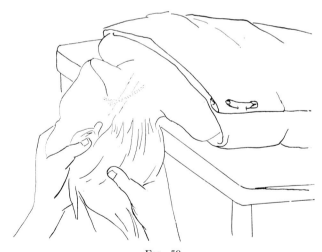

FIG. 59
Position of child for jugular vein puncture

applied to the puncture while the child is in the sitting position. When the nurse has ascertained that there is no bleeding, pressure is released and the child can be returned to his bed.

REQUIREMENTS. As for venepuncture.

PUNCTURE OF THE FEMORAL VEIN

This is another method by which blood may be obtained from an infant or a small child. Care must be taken to ensure cleanliness of the inguinal and perineal regions to avoid contamination due to urine or faeces.

The child is placed on a flat, firm table. The legs are abducted so as to expose the inguinal region. The child is held firmly to prevent any movement. After the needle has been removed, firm pressure must be applied for 3-5 minutes.

REQUIREMENTS. As for venepuncture.

ADMINISTRATION OF FLUIDS

The maintenance of body fluids is of primary importance in the treatment of disease. Usually, the alimentary tract provides the means of adequate food and water intake. In some diseases the normal means of supplying the needs of the body has to be replaced or supplemented by parenteral feeding. Dehydration and loss of electrolytes occurs very rapidly in infants suffering from severe vomiting and diarrhoea, toxaemic shock, intestinal obstruction and other disturbances of electrolyte and acid/base balance. There are several routes by which water, protein and electrolytes can be adjusted. Those most widely used include:

1. Intravenous.
2. Subcutaneous.

Intravenous Route

The majority of infusions are by the intravenous route. It is the most efficient means of giving fluid and electrolytes as well as proteins, but it is not without dangers. It must be carefully controlled and adjusted to the individual child's needs. Renal function is depressed during sleep so that when it is continued during the night, adjustment to the flow and amount may have to be made by the doctor. The type of fluid to be given is dependent on the condition for which it is required. Fluids used for replacement include: plasma, whole blood, packed cells, amino acids in

5 per cent glucose and electrolyte solutions; e.g., Dextrose solution, Saline solution, Saline dextrose, Sodium lactate.

There are two methods used; (a) Venepuncture and (b) Venesection. Some of the requirements vary in each type but the control, maintenance and nursing care are the same in both methods.

VENEPUNCTURE

A needle or cannula is inserted via the skin directly into a vein and is preferred to venesection (cutting down). It is used whenever possible, but difficulty may be encountered in infants and young children, especially if they are in a collapsed state or severely dehydrated.

REQUIREMENTS:

Sterile equipment:
1. Swabs.
2. Skin cleansing lotion.
3. Needles: intracatheter or Batemann's needles.
4. Bowl with saline.
5. 5 ml. syringe.

Additional equipment:
6. Giving set—infant type disposable set.
7. Flask of fluid to be given.
8. Flask of normal saline.
9. Gauge label (if required).
10. Splint.
11. Bandages, adhesive tape.
12. Water repellent sheet.
13. Receptacle for disposable items.
14. Receptacle for salvage.
15. Infusion stand.

PREPARATION OF THE CHILD. A simple explanation should be given to the older child if he is well enough. This will help him to understand what is about to happen and will also ensure his co-operation in keeping his arm as still as possible. Sedation may be necessary if the child is apprehensive and restless. The child is made comfortable and the clothes are removed from the limb. A prepared splint of the correct size is applied to the arm, taking care that the adhesive tape is not applied too tightly which might

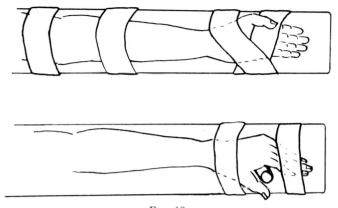

FIG. 60

Immobilisation of arm—note position of adhesive tape

constrict the blood vessels and interfere with the circulation of the injected fluid (Fig. 60). In the younger child it may be necessary to splint or tie the other arm to prevent him touching or pulling the needle out (Fig. 42 or Fig. 62).

The doctor then inserts the needle or intracatheter and the filled and prepared giving set is fitted to the needle. A swab is placed over the needle insertion and held in position with a strip of adhesive tape; care must be taken not to encircle the limb and constrict the circulation.

VENESECTION

When fluids are urgently required and difficulty is encountered in entering a vein by venepuncture, a vein must be exposed surgically. A small incision is made into the vein and a cannula or polyethylene tubing inserted. In infants, the site chosen is usually the internal saphenous vein of the lower limb and it has the advantage that it can be used 2 or 3 times if necessary (Fig. 61). In

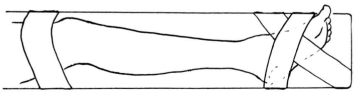

FIG. 61

Immobilisation of leg—note position of adhesive tape

older children, the median basilic vein of the upper limb is the usual one of choice.

REQUIREMENTS:

Trolley with sterile equipment on upper shelf:
1. Swabs.
2. Skin cleansing lotions.
3. Polythene tubing, Portex intravenous cannulae or Batemann's needles.
4. Bowl for saline.
5. 5 ml. and 1 ml. syringes and hypodermic needles.
6. Catgut 3/0 and black silk 3/0.
7. *Instruments:*
    Bard-Parker handle and blades.
    2 fine dissecting forceps.
    1 aneurism needle.
    1 probe.
    1 pr. dressing scissors.
    1 pr. fine pointed scissors.
    2 prs. Mosquito forceps.
    1 pr. Spencer Wells forceps.
    1 needle holding forceps
    Skin suture needles.

If the infusion is for a baby having small amounts of fluid ½-hourly, or when drugs are being given, the following will be required:
Heller's valve.
3-way adaptor.
10 ml. or 20 ml. syringe.

Trolley—lower shelf:
1. Disposable giving set (with measured chamber).
2. Flask of fluid to be given with bottle hanger.
3. Flask of normal saline.
4. Splints, bandages, adhesive tape.
5. Local anaesthesia.
6. Gauge label for the flask (if necessary).
7. Receptacle for used instruments.
8. Receptacle for salvage.

9. Receptacle for disposable items.
10. Bedcage.

In addition: Anglepoise lamp and a stand for intravenous infusion.

PREPARATION OF THE CHILD. A simple explanation to the older child if he is well enough will help him to understand what is about to happen and why he should keep still. He will accept the situation and not be alarmed at the proceedings if he is well prepared. The smaller child or the very ill child may become restless and it is therefore wiser if sedation is given before the procedure is carried out.

The nurse prepares the splint, which should be of the correct size, and if the lower limb is to be used she straps the splint to the limb exposing the inner malleolus. Care should be taken not to constrict the blood vessels, which might interfere with the circulation of the fluid injected. The splint is then tied securely to the bed. The other leg is immobilised by applying a strip of lint round the ankle as protective padding and holding it in position with a bandage. This can be most safely accomplished by making a clove hitch over the lint and tying the ends around the side of the bed (Fig. 62). A slip knot should never be used because it

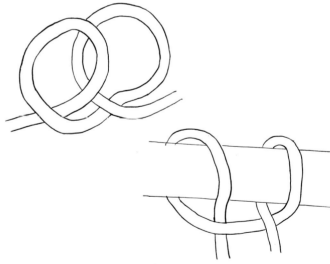

FIG. 62
Clove hitch for use as restraint

can easily cause constriction of the limb when pulled with the movement of the limb. All methods of immobilisation should be inspected two hourly and re-applied if necessary. A woollen sock may be put on this foot. The child should be kept warm and only the area required exposed. If the extremities are cold, the blood vessels will contract making the process of setting up the infusion much more difficult.

After the doctor has inserted the needle and sutured the skin and a dressing has been applied, the child is made comfortable. A small cage is placed between the bedclothes and the limb. If a conventional type of infusion set and a graduated vacolitre flask is used, the amount to be given should be clearly marked on the gauge label which is attached to the flask. The infant disposable set allows a reasonably accurate regulation of the amount of fluid to be given over a given period of time. It consists of a graduated burette chamber which is filled with the amount of fluid the child is to receive. The flow control clamps adjust the rate of flow through the paediatric drip in the drip chamber which is metered to provide approximately 60 drops per minute.

The type of fluid and the amount is written on the prescription sheet by the doctor.

While the infusion is in progress, the child must be observed carefully.

The following points are important :

1. Leakage at the site of insertion may occur. This may be due to:
   (*a*) Fluid entering the tissues. The first indication of this may be the presence of oedema surrounding the site of insertion. For this reason it is important not to bandage over the site of insertion. This part can be covered with a sterile swab which is loosely held in position with a strip of adhesive tape. An older child may complain of pain and the rate of the infusion flow decrease. The doctor should be notified at once and if the infusion is to be continued, the nurse will have to prepare for another venesection or venepuncture.
   (*b*) It may be due to faulty connection which should be remedied by the doctor. A small tray containing sterile swabs, adhesive tape, and sterile petroleum jelly to seal the connecting parts, should be prepared.

2. The infusion may stop due to blockage of the needle or cannula. The doctor is notified immediately and a tray prepared, containing the following sterile equipment:

1. Bowl for normal saline.
2. Flask of normal saline.
3. 5 ml. or 10 ml. syringe.
4. Flask of sterile sodium citrate.
5. Swabs.
6. Adhesive tape.

3. The rate of flow may be decreased or stopped for a variety of reasons:

(a) Spasms of the vein due to mechanical irritation; i.e., entry of a needle or cannula into the vein, or due to cold.

(b) Due to abnormal position of the limb; e.g., if the child bends the knee or flexes the arm for any length of time. The height of the flask as well as the pressure from the clamp will determine the rate of flow.

(c) Adhesive tape may be too tight, leading to constriction of blood vessels.

If the flow does not resume immediately, the doctor should be notified.

4. An accurate fluid balance chart must be kept. This chart should contain all measured amounts of fluids given and all output.

5. The bottle must never be allowed to empty completely, so the level of the fluid in the flask should be watched constantly. Failure to observe this may lead to the introduction of air into the circulation.

6. The new vacolitre bottle should be checked by two people to ensure that the correct fluid is given.

7. While the infusion is in progress, oral fluids may be discontinued. Salivary secretions are diminished or suppressed, therefore care of the mouth is essential.

8. The child should be made comfortable and his position changed to avoid interference with the blood supply at pressure areas, and also to prevent respiratory complications. The infant is kept warm, but overheating should be avoided. The napkin is changed frequently and the buttocks washed in the normal manner.

9. Any signs of generalised oedema, respiratory distress, and convulsions, must be reported at once.

COMPLETION OF THE INTRAVENOUS INFUSION. When the infusion has been completed, the nurse prepares the following tray:

Sterile equipment:
1. Swabs.
2. Container with skin cleansing lotion.
3. 1 pr. stitch scissors.
   1 pr. dissecting forceps.

Additional equipment:
4. 2 in. bandage and adhesive tape.
5. Receptacle for disposable items.
6. Receptacle for instruments.

The infusion is discontinued by closing the control clip and, using aseptic technique, the needle or polythene tubing is removed. The area is cleaned and a sterile swab is applied. After the splint has been removed, the sutured area is bandaged, and the child is made comfortable. Stitches are usually removed on the fifth day.

SCALP VEIN INFUSION

This procedure is performed on infants up to six months of age. The superficial scalp veins in infants are more prominent, thus permitting easy entry into the vein and thereby avoiding the necessity of using a larger vein for venesection. It is an excellent method of giving fluids.

REQUIREMENTS:

Trolley with sterile equipment on upper shelf:
1. 2 containers for skin cleansing lotions.
2. Foil tray containing:
   (*a*) Special scalp vein needles, various sizes.
   (*b*) Polythene tubing, polythene adaptor or disposable scalp vein set.
3. Swabs.
4. Container with normal saline.
5. Giving set.

Lower shelf:
6. Vacolitres of sterile fluids for infusion.
7. Adhesive tape (cut into 4-5-inch narrow strips).

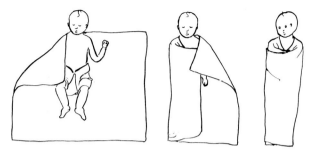

Fig. 63

Immobilisation of infant using blanket. Note how the
blanket is taken well over shoulders.

8. Bandages.
9. Arm splints.
10. Covered sandbags or Sorbo rubber sections to immobilise
    the head.
11. Infusion stand.

PREPARATION OF THE CHILD. The infant's scalp is shaved at
the area chosen for the puncture. The temporal veins on either
side are most frequently chosen. The child is wrapped in a shawl

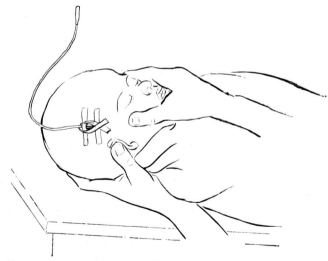

Fig. 64

Position of child for scalp vein transfusion

or blanket (Fig. 63) and if necessary the arms are restrained with splints. If the child is liable to be restless, sedation such as chloral hydrate may be ordered, and should be given at least 30 minutes before the procedure is due to begin. The infant's head is held gently but firmly to one side with the prepared side uppermost. Once the infusion is running, sandbags or Sorbo rubber sections may be used to maintain the position and prevent excessive movement of the head (Fig. 64).

While the infusion is running in, the following points must be noted:

1. A certain amount of movement is permissible but the infant should not be allowed to become restless.

2. The infusion site must be watched carefully because these veins are superficial and small. It may happen that the needle penetrates through the wall of the vessel allowing escape of fluid into the adjacent tissue leading to swelling. Should this happen the infusion must be clamped off, the doctor notified and a new venepuncture prepared for.

3. For the observation and care of the child having fluids administered intravenously, see venesection.

4. When the infusion is completed and the needle is withdrawn, firm pressure on the punctured site is necessary to avoid oozing and loss of blood. A small haematoma readily occurs if this is not done.

BLOOD TRANSFUSION

INDICATIONS FOR BLOOD TRANSFUSIONS. In general, there are two main reasons for blood transfusions:

1. To restore the volume of circulating blood as in haemorrhage; where a long and extensive operation is to be performed blood must be replaced.

2. To provide some cellular or protein component which is deficient in the particular patient;
   e.g. (*a*) red cells as in hypochromic anaemia, haemolytic anaemia and leukaemia.
   (*b*) platelets in thrombocytopaenia or deficiency in the coagulation factor, as in haemophilia and haemorrhagic disease of the newborn.

TYPES OF BLOOD AVAILABLE.
1. *Whole blood.* A standard bottle contains approximately 540 ml. of citrated blood.
2. *'Maximum survival blood'.* Whole blood less than seven days after donation.
3. *'Fresh blood'.* Whole blood as fresh as possible and within a few hours of donation.
4. *Concentrated red cells.* One bottle contains the red cells obtained from two bottles of whole blood plus some plasma.
5. *Washed concentrated red cells.* One bottle contains the red cells obtained from two bottles of 'maximum survival whole blood' suspended in saline, the plasma having been removed completely. (Used for special cases of haemolytic anaemia.)
6. *'Platelet rich' whole blood.* Fresh blood is collected using siliconised apparatus and bottle in order to preserve platelet activity.

CARE OF THE BLOOD. Blood should not normally be warmed before transfusion. Overheating causes disintegration of red blood cells. The only exception is where the blood is to be given to an infant for an exchange transfusion. The bottle containing the blood should be placed in water at a temperature of 40°C (100°F), the temperature of the water being checked constantly with a thermometer.

CHECKING THE BOTTLE. The label on the bottle must be checked carefully before the blood is given to the child. The label must contain the child's name, ward, blood group, and Rhesus type. Blood and blood products must be regarded as potentially dangerous fluids and great care must be taken to ensure that the correct bottle of blood is given to the correct patient.

CARE OF THE CHILD. The child should be propped up in bed, made comfortable and kept warm, but not overheated. When the transfusion is for a child suffering from haemorrhage he is nursed in the head-low position. Excessive warming must be avoided in cases of haemorrhage, since this may remove the compensatory constriction of the peripheral blood vessels and cause a fall in blood pressure. Special care of the mouth will be required, if oral fluids are not permitted. The child's position should be changed to avoid interference with the blood supply to the pressure areas. In infants, the napkin is changed frequently, the buttocks being washed in the normal manner.

Throughout the transfusion careful supervision is essential to minimise the adverse effects of a reaction. An accurate record must be kept on the fluid intake and output. Should any of the following signs present themselves, medical aid must be summoned:

1. Increase in pulse rate: should the pulse rate increase by more than 20 per minute.
2. Rise in temperature.
3. Complaints of headache, nausea and of feeling cold.
4. Rigor.
5. Inadequate urinary output.
6. Urticaria due to allergic reaction.
7. Respiratory distress; e.g., dyspnoea, cyanosis, collapse.
8. Jaundice.
9. Convulsions.

When a transfusion is continued for several days, the giving set will require to be changed to avoid the possibility of micro-organisms multiplying within the lumen of the tube. It is also advisable to change to a fresh giving set whenever a transfusion of blood is preceded or followed by an infusion of dextrose solution. Red blood corpuscles tend to agglutinate in a high concentration of dextrose and such cells may then be haemolysed in the patient.

On completion of the transfusion, the empty bottles must not be washed and are kept in the ward for at least 24 hours after use. Details of the transfusion are entered on a special form and any untoward reactions can then be traced without any difficulty.

EXCHANGE TRANSFUSION

REASON. Exchange transfusion is an operation when 90 per cent of the patient's circulating blood is withdrawn and replaced by donor blood. Originally, it was developed for the treatment of haemolytic disease of the newborn which was due to rhesus incompatibility but it may also be considered in conditions such as:

A B O incompatibility or other haemolytic conditions where the serum bilirubin concentration rises to 18-20 mg. per 100 ml., and also in cases of severe poisoning.

Exchange transfusion is carried out with whole blood or packed cells. When it is performed on an infant suffering from haemolytic disease of the newborn due to rhesus incompatibility, rhesus negative blood of suitable group is used. In most cases the umbilical vein is cannulated but occasionally the umbilical vein is unsuitable for performing the exchange transfusion, and a vene-section is carried out on the femoral vein or an arm vein.

PREPARATION OF THE CHILD. As soon as the ward is notified of the impending admission, a cot is prepared and heated with clothing placed in readiness. A tray is prepared for a fontanelle tap to obtain blood for bilirubin test, Coomb's test and cross matching. The umbilical cord is redressed; either a dry dressing or a saline dressing is applied. For a saline dressing the following items will be required:

1. Swabs.
2. Container for warm normal saline.
3. Jaconet and crepe bandage.
4. Receptacle for disposable items.

ON ADMISSION. The infant is weighed and measured. The umbilical cord is dressed with a swab soaked in warmed normal saline or a dry swab, and is covered with jaconet and a crepe band-age. Care must be taken to avoid bandaging too tightly. The saline dressing is applied so that the cord is kept moist and patent for the introduction of the polythene tubing into the umbilical vein. The infant is then dressed in warm clothing and placed in the prepared cot.

REQUIREMENTS:

Trolley with sterile equipment on upper shelf:

1. Swabs.
2. Bowl for normal saline.
3. Containers for (*a*) heparin solution.
                 (*b*) cleansing solution.
4. 2 ml. syringe and No. 1 needles.
5. 3 × 10 ml. syringes or 3 × 20 ml. Henderson's syringes (Fig. 65).
6. 3-way adaptors.
7. 3 nozzles adaptors and rubber washers (for Henderson's syringe).
8. 1 × 4- foot length rubber tubing.
9. *Instruments:*
   1 Bard-Parker handle and blade.
   1 pr. stitch scissors.
   1 pr. iris scissors.
   2 prs. Mosquito forceps.

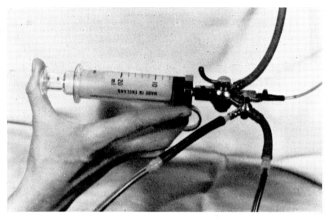

Fig. 65

Henderson's exchange syringe, showing attachments for heparinised saline, blood for replacement, umbilical catheter and waste blood.

2 prs. curved pressure forceps.

1 pr. small dissecting forceps.

Aneurism needle.

Cord ligatures.

4 towel clips

Atraumatic catgut 3/0 on a curved cutting needle.

10. 1 Portex No. 9 umbilical catheter.
11. 1 Jacques disposable catheter No. 14 and 1 Portex feeding catheter.
12. 2 large towels with a centrehole.
13. Sterile towels, gowns and gloves.

Lower shelf :

1. Padded T-splint or wooden rectangle covered with foam.
2. Bandage and gamgee tissue for the infant.
3. 1 crepe bandage or strips of Velcro.
4. Elastoplast.
5. 2 disposable intravenous giving set.
6. 2 bottles normal saline.
7. Flasks of blood.
8. 1 vial Heparin 10,000 units per ml.
9. 1 vial Calcium gluconate 10 per cent.
10. 1 bottle of 8·4 per cent Sod. bicarbonate.

11. Waste bucket.
12. Bowl of cold water with biotergic—for soaking instruments.
13. Intravenous infusion stand.
14. Stethoscope.
15. Record chart and holder, pen, watch with seconds hand.
16. Receptacle for salvage.
17. Receptacle for disposable items.
18. Receptacle for instruments.

Additional equipment:

Resuscitation tray.
Suction apparatus with suction ends and catheters.

CARE OF THE INFANT. The room should be warm about 30°C or 86°F and a good light available. The infant is undressed but bootees and gloves are kept on. The arms, legs and chest are protected with gamgee tissue and the infant is bandaged on to the T-splint, leaving the abdominal area exposed. Alternatively, the infant is placed on a foam covered wooden board and the limbs

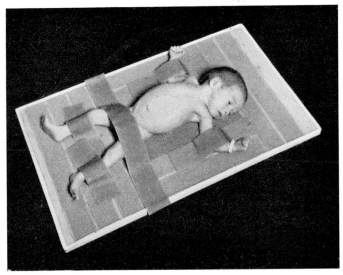

FIG. 66
Infant immobilising board. (By kind permission of Down Bros. and
Mayer & Phelps Ltd.)

are immobilised with strips of Velcro, which are fixed to the board with strong adhesive tape. This board fits most types of incubators (Fig. 66). A light cotton blanket is placed over the lower extremities and covered hot water bottles may be placed at either side of the child. To prevent the infant from crying, a teat soaked in rose hip syrup and filled with a sterile swab, may be given to him to suck.

The nurse is responsible for keeping an accurate record of the time and the amount of blood withdrawn and replaced. The infant's pulse is felt and counted and the respiration rate checked regularly. Any irregularities in pulse rate and any respiratory distress must be reported at once. The amount of blood withdrawn and replaced depends on the weight of the infant. On completion of the transfusion, the catheter is left in position and enclosed in a dry sterile swab, ready for another exchange transfusion should the bilirubin be increased after subsequent blood tests.

AFTER CARE OF THE INFANT. The infant is taken off the T-splint, or wooden board, redressed, and may be placed in an oxygen tent. Fluids may not be given for 6-8 hours. Although it is important to keep the infant warm, overheating must be avoided. The baby's general condition, his pulse rate, respiration and temperature, should be carefully observed for several hours.

SUBCUTANEOUS INFUSION, OR HYPODERMOCLYSIS

This method of giving fluid to correct dehydration and salt loss is used for an infant when a small quantity is required, which cannot adequately be given orally, and the intravenous route is deemed unnecessary. It is a useful method to resort to where a small infant has had repeated intravenous infusions, and it is considered wise to avoid another venesection.

PRINCIPLES INVOLVED. The use of an isotonic solution, i.e. one that has the same sodium chloride concentration as that of tissue fluids. The fluid when given into the subcutaneous tissues can be satisfactorily absorbed, providing the speed of flow is not too great.

The Use of Hyaluronidase. This is a tissue enzyme which is a spreading factor causing breakdown of the collagen fibres in tissues, thus permitting the fluid to spread over a much wider area and, therefore, be more readily absorbed.

REQUIREMENTS:

Trolley containing sterile equipment on upper shelf:
1, Gauze swabs and wool balls.
2. Containers for cleansing lotions.
3. Instruments:
  2 prs. dressing forceps for skin cleansing.
  2 twelve-inch lengths rubber tubing with adaptors.
  1 'Y' connection. 2 screw clips.
  2 No. 12 or No. 1 needles, or special subcutaneous needles.
  2 ml. syringe with No. 12 needle for hyaluronidase.
  2 dressing towels.

Lower shelf:
1. Flask of normal saline or fluid to be given and graduated label.
2. Disposable giving set.
3. Ampoule of hyaluronidase and sterile water.
4. File.
5. Nobecutane.
6. Receptacle for salvage.
7. Receptacle for disposable items.
8. Safety pins.
9. Cotton blanket.
10. Suitable restraints for infant.

At bedside :
Anglepoise lamp.
Intravenous infusion stand.

PREPARATION OF PATIENT. The infant is suitably restrained and the chosen site exposed. The site which can be used with most safety and ease is the outer middle one-third of each thigh. Each ankle can be restrained with a clove hitch to the foot of the bed. If this site has been used recently and an alternative has to be found, the chest wall can be used, inserting the needle approximately $1\frac{1}{2}$ inches out from the nipple line. Nearer the axilla is too danger-ous. It is difficult to restrain the arms and the needles may easily penetrate too far. The subscapular region is another alternative. The infant lies on his face, and the needles are inserted just below the lower border of each scapula. For either of these last two sites, it is necessary to restrain both wrists and ankles very carefully.

METHOD. Two nurses are required; one to perform the procedure and the second to assist with equipment and comfort the
infant. Both nurses wash and dry their hands carefully. The
assistant prepares short lengths of strapping to fix the needle and
tubing adequately, and prepares the infant. The performer assembles the apparatus, the flask is hung from the stand, and all air
eliminated; the tubing is then firmly clamped. The needles and
end of tubing from the 'Y' connection are left on the instrument

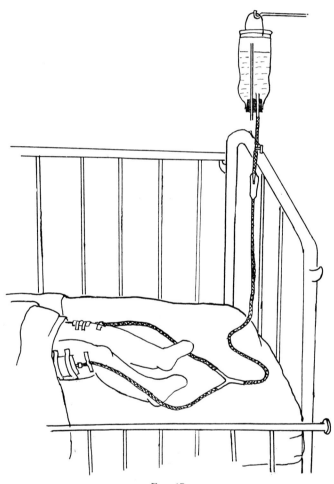

FIG. 67
Subcutaneous infusion

tray and the needles covered with a swab. Hyaluronidase is drawn up ready in the syringe. One ampoule of 3,000 units is divided between two sites. The skin area is carefully cleansed and dried. Dressing towels are placed in position with a minimal area of skin exposed. The needles and tubing are then transferred on to the towel, and the needles inserted subcutaneously into the chosen site. The needle should be inserted approximately two-thirds of its length at an angle of 15° and it is strapped into position before the second needle is inserted (Fig. 67). Once both are secure, the clamps are removed and, providing the fluid is flowing satisfactorily, the hyaluronidase is injected into both ends of tubing just above the needles. The screw clips are adjusted so that the flow is at the prescribed rate. It may be desirable to give 90 ml. into both sites within one hour, or less may be ordered to be given each hour over a longer period. The rate of flow must not exceed the rate of absorption and induration should not be allowed to develop. Some oedema will be present but this should be soft and obviously dispersing. The area should be neither unduly red nor blanched. The rate of flow can be altered as desired; if necessary one side may be clamped off until the fluid has dispersed.

On completion of the appropriate amount being given, the needles are withdrawn and a small nobecutane soaked swab applied. The restrainers are removed and the baby left warmly wrapped up.

While the infusion is in progress, it is not essential that a nurse stays with the infant, providing he is adequately restrained. It is important to ensure that the baby is kept warm; a cage should be placed in the bed; the area must be examined at intervals, and the flow regulated as necessary. Leakage or induration must be reported immediately.

BONE MARROW PUNCTURE

REASON. This procedure is indicated to aid the diagnosis of blood dyscrasias such as leukaemia, reticuloendotheliosis, and to obtain cultures. A small amount of marrow juice is withdrawn from the iliac crest, sternum or tibia. The tissue is examined for cellular structure.

PREPARATION OF THE CHILD. This is a painful and unpleasant procedure. Every precaution should be taken that the child does not see the procedure or the instruments used. Sedation is usually given before the procedure is due to begin. The nurse places the child on a firm surface, such as a table, and gently restrains the child to prevent any movement taking place. The position of the child will depend on the choice of the site to be punctured.

(a) Sternum: The child is placed in the recumbent position.

(b) Crest of iliac: Recumbent position, the pelvis slightly raised on the side to be punctured.

(c) Tibia: In small infants a splint may be applied to the limb to give adequate support in order to avoid fracture of the bone. This may occur when force is used to introduce the needle.

When the procedure is completed and the needle withdrawn, firm pressure must be applied to prevent bleeding. The child is then lifted carefully back into his bed and made comfortable.

REQUIREMENTS:

Trolley with sterile equipment on upper shelf:

1. 3 containers for skin cleansing lotions.
2. Swabs.
3. 20 ml. syringe and 2 ml. syringe, needles No. 17 and No. 12.
4. Packet containing bone puncture needles.
5. Dissecting forceps for cleansing skin.
6. Sterile towels, gowns and gloves.

Lower shelf:

7. Receptacle for disposable items.
8. Receptacle for used instruments.
9. Local anaesthesia.
10. Adhesive tape.
11. Nobecutane.
12. Resuscitation tray.

SPECIAL TRAY FOR THE ASSISTANT DOCTOR OR LABORATORY TECHNICIAN:

1. Fine untoothed dissecting forceps.
2. 6 clean slides.
3. 4 watch glasses.
4. Fixing fluid.
5. Lables.

BIBLIOGRAPHY

Barrie, H. & Harris, R. (1963). Exchange transfusion theory and practice. *Nurs. Times*, **59**, 1264, 1317.

Blackburn, E. K. (1966). Indications for blood transfusion. *Nurs. Times*, 62, 592.

Fuerst, E. V. & Wolff, L. (1967). *Fundamentals of Nursing*, 3rd ed., Unit 14, Part 39. Philadelphia: Lippincott.

Kessel, J. (1967). *The Essentials of Paediatrics for Nurses*, 3rd ed. Edinburgh: Livingstone.

Oppé, T. E. (1961). *Modern Textbook of Paediatrics for Nurses. Exchange Transfusion.* London: Heinemann.

Portex Rossiter Set (1962). *Nurs. Times*, **58**, 179.

Tovey, G. H. (1967). Nursing care during blood transfusion. *Nurs. Mirror*, **124**, 2, 35.

CHAPTER XVI

RADIOLOGICAL PROCEDURES

Barium swallow and meal; barium enema; tracheo-oesophageal investigations; air encephalography; excretion pyelogram; bronchography; cardiac catheterisation.

D IAGNOSTIC X-ray examinations and investigations are essential for the diagnosis and control of treatment of many diseases in infancy and childhood.

Although no X-ray examination should be withheld which might be of possible value, it is important that reduction of hazards by ionising radiations should be always borne in mind, because infants and children are more vulnerable than adults to such risks. The gonads of the patient should be covered with a suitable lead shield whenever possible and fluoroscopy or screening reduced to a minimum.

Within a reasonable time, all paediatric clinics should have image intensifiers installed and when this is combined with the use of closed circuit television, the use of standard fluoroscopes should cease. Not only do image intensifiers reduce the radiation dose, but they always permit screening to take place in a lighted room so avoiding the apprehension caused by examinations conducted in total, or almost total, darkness.

Nurses assisting in radiological procedure should wear suitable protective aprons. When they assist in the handling or positioning of the child protective gloves should also be worn. In order to reduce radiation hazards to a minimum, the nursing staff involved in X-ray procedure should be changed at intervals in order to avoid the same nurse being continuously exposed to radiation. It must be understood, that with modern protective devices in X-ray departments, there is no risk involved to any individual working in a diagnostic X-ray room, and the staff will not be exposed to any harm by ionising radiations.

BARIUM SWALLOW AND MEAL

REASON. These examinations are carried out to aid diagnosis

when there is a suspected abnormality of the alimentary tract. The following are some of the conditions which may be diagnosed by findings after a swallow or meal—hiatus hernia, oesophageal stricture or diverticulum, oesophageal varices, pyloric stenosis, peptic ulcers and hairballs in the stomach.

PRINCIPLES INVOLVED. Barium sulphate is an opaque medium, non-toxic and is not absorbed. Because of its opacity to X-rays, it clearly shows the size, position and shape of the stomach, together with the character of peristaltic waves. The rate at which the barium leaves the stomach and any irregularities of contour caused by ulceration or new growth will be visible.

PREPARATION OF THE CHILD. The child should have no food for four hours prior to the examination. Suitable clothing, either a cotton or woollen garment without buttons, should be worn. Adequate explanation about the dim lights is essential for the older child. The smaller or apprehensive child should always be accompanied by his mother or a nurse he knows, and she should not leave him during the proceedings.

REQUIREMENTS:

1. Barium. This is prepared according to instructions but is usually not diluted for barium swallow.
2. Cup and spoon, or bottle with a large holed teat.
3. Bib.

METHOD:

(a) BARIUM SWALLOW. The barium is given to drink while the lights are dimmed and the child is in position on the table. The progress of the barium is watched through the X-ray screen. X-rays are then taken as required.

(b) BARIUM MEAL. As soon as the barium has been swallowed, its progress is watched through the X-ray screen and pictures are taken at suitable moments. Instructions will be given by the radiographer as to the times subsequent X-rays will be required. These may be taken over a period of hours.

Cardiac Investigation

When the oesophagus is outlined during barium swallow, the degree of cardiac enlargement is clearly defined, and for this reason a barium swallow may be ordered prior to cardiac investigations. It is not necessary for the child to fast in preparation for this examination.

INVESTIGATIONS FOR TRACHEO-OESOPHAGEAL ABNORMALITY

REASON: Examinations are carried out where there is a suspected tracheo-oesophageal fistula with or without oesophageal atresia or an oesophageal atresia.

To diagnose a suspected tracheo-oesophageal fistula a viscid contrast medium propyliodone may be used. This substance does not irritate the respiratory tract. Oesophageal atresia is diagnosed by the passage of an opaque catheter (Fig. 68).

PREPARATION AND CARE OF THE CHILD. The infant may be in an incubator, in which case this is transported to the X-ray department. Otherwise, he is warmly wrapped up and taken to the department by a nurse. The infant should be dressed in loose woollen, or cotton garments without buttons; also mittens and bootees to prevent chilling during the procedure.

The possibliity of aspiration of saliva must be constantly borne in mind. Such infants should not be left without a nurse and the position which is considered most safe must be maintained. Alternatives are to keep the infant with his head low and to the side, preventing saliva accumulating in the mouth, or keep the infant upright allowing drainage of saliva down into the pouch of the oesophagus. The saliva is aspirated from the pouch through a fine catheter which is left in position.

REQUIREMENTS:

Sterile equipment:
1. Spoon.
2. 2 ml. syringe and withdrawing needle.
3. Oesophageal catheter 9 F.G. or 4 E.G. or radio opaque catheter.
4. Mucus extractor or suction equipment.

Additional equipment :
5. Warmed ampoule of propyliodone.
6. Paper tissues.
7. Receptacle for salvage.
8. Receptacle for disposable items.

METHOD. Normally this examination is performed under

screening when the infant is given about 1-2 ml. of the contrast
medium to swallow from a spoon. The lights are put out and the
progress of the medium is watched under the screen. An alternative method is to lubricate the oesophageal catheter with the

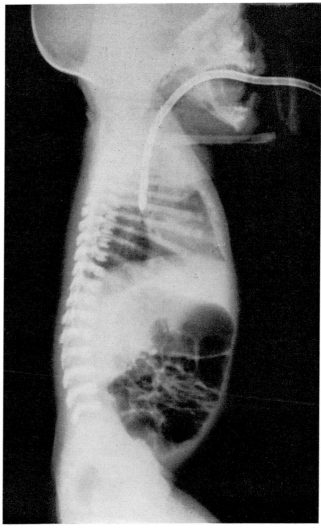

Fig. 68
Radio opaque catheter demonstrating an eosophageal atresia

medium and gently pass it, watching the progress under screening, or to use a radio opaque catheter.

AFTER CARE OF THE CHILD. If an atresia, or obstruction of the oesophagus is present, the medium should be sucked out before returning to the ward. This is to prevent further complications of this condition. The most effective method of aspiration is with direct vision when the endoscope is passed by an anaesthetist and any material removed through an open-ended catheter attached to a strong suction machine.

GASTROGRAFIN

This is a contrast medium for radiological investigation of the gastro-intestinal tract. It may be given orally, or as an enema. It is an aqueous solution and is much more rapidly dispersed, reaching the colon in a small infant in under one hour. It is, therefore, of use in suspected obstruction and in intestinal atresia.

Very small quantities are required. In an infant weighing 3·2 kg. or 7 lb., 10 ml. given orally will reach the rectum in forty-five minutes. When given rectally more is required and the medium is diluted 1 in 4 parts of water.

Requirements and preparation for the infant are the same as those for tracheo-oesophageal investigations. There is no specific after care.

BARIUM ENEMA

REASONS AND PRINCIPLES. This X-ray examination is also an aid to diagnosis. It will outline any abnormality of contour or of emptying of the lower bowel, such as occurs in Hirschsprung's disease, or idiopathic megacolon (Fig. 69).

PREPARATION OF THE CHILD. Instructions must be obtained from the doctor in charge. For children with suspected megacolon, whether congenital or acquired, no prior preparation of the bowel may be desired before barium enema as any purgations may alter the outline and mobility of the bowel. Infants and young children who are very apprehensive should be adequately sedated prior to examination to prevent resistance to retrograde injection of barium and to prevent the expulsion of the enema.

The mother or a nurse known to the child should always accompany and stay with the younger child. She can do much to allay fear and permit the examination to be carried out quickly and with the least unpleasantness. The older child requires adequate explanation and someone from the ward to accompany him if he is at all apprehensive.

On the morning of examination, the normal diet is given. The child is dressed for transfer to the X-ray department.

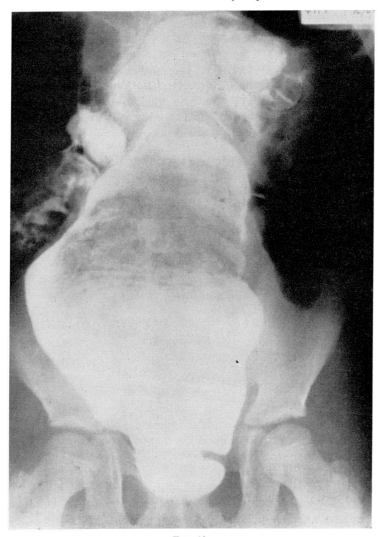

FIG. 69
Barium enema demonstrating Hirschsprung's disease
P.N.P.—K

REQUIREMENTS:

1. Tray as for enema.
2. Barium sulphate mixed with normal saline to prevent the possibility of water intoxication in cases of megacolon— temperature 37·2°C or 99°F.
3. Bedpan and cover, or readily accessible toilet facilities.

METHOD. The enema is given under screening and the progress watched. The barium is syphoned back after X-ray.

AFTER CARE OF THE CHILD. On return to the ward, a bowel action is encouraged. If all the barium is not returned, it may form solid lumps, which can be extremely difficult to remove. Dioctyl-medo, a detergent lubricant drug, has been found of value in removing inspissated faeces and barium.

ALTERNATIVE TO BARIUM ENEMA FOR CONSTIPATION OR FAECAL SOILING

Constipation or faecal soiling may be investigated by barium follow-through examination after adequate purgation. At least two days of purgation is required, which is followed by barium sulphate by mouth in four divided doses given the next day. X-rays are taken the following morning to show the size of the colon. Subsequent films are arranged to assess the rate of emptying. This method has the advantage that it can be done while attending as an outpatient.

SIALOGRAM

REASON. This is an X-ray examination of the parotid duct carried out in suspected blockage due to infection, or calculus, and to outline the salivary ducts in cases of sialectasis. Opaque medium is injected along the duct and X-rays taken in an endeavour to outline it, or define the blockage.

CARE OF THE CHILD. This is not a painful procedure, but can be difficult and certainly impossible with a frightened and struggling child. Suitable sedation may, therefore, have to be given at the appropriate time beforehand. Adequate explanation is given to the older child and a nurse known to the child should be present throughout.

METHOD. It is necessary for the child to lie quite still with his mouth open. Once the parotid duct is located beside the molar teeth, the opaque medium is injected. The mouth is thoroughly swabbed to remove any excess media, which might give a false picture when X-rays are taken. The use of a mouth gag is frightening and should be avoided if at all possible. A mouth wash is given after the proceedings are over.

AIR ENCEPHALOGRAPHY AND VENTRICULOGRAPHY

This procedure is carried out to obtain an X-ray film of the cerebral ventricles. A lumbar puncture is made, cerebrospinal fluid is withdrawn, and air is injected. The X-ray (positive) will show lighter areas corresponding to the ventricles. The shape, size and position of the ventricles may give valuable information as to the position of tumours in the cranial cavity, or in an existing hydrocephalus, the degree of dilation of the ventricles.

REQUIREMENTS. The same requirements as for lumbar puncture, and in addition:

1. 100 ml. measure for cerebro-spinal fluid.
2. 20 ml. syringe.
3. Extra pillows if necessary.
4. Vomit bowl.
5. Resuscitation trolley (Chapter XX).

PREPARATION AND CARE OF THE CHILD. The child is prepared as for a general anaesthesia. He may either be heavily sedated or a general anaesthetic is given. He is positioned sitting upright well supported with pillows. The head should be resting on the pillows ensuring a clear airway. A lumbar puncture is performed and the amount of fluid withdrawn is replaced by air. The amount varies with the age of the child.

The whole procedure can be carried out in the X-ray department, but if the lumbar puncture is carried out in the ward, it is important that there are no delays in transporting the child to the X-ray department and that he is kept in the upright position during this time. The head must not be allowed to fall sideways or on to the chest.

Throughout the procedure it is important to watch for early signs of shock or distress. Collapse may occur quite suddenly and is due to the change of intracranial pressure. The child should be laid flat immediately and oxygen administered.

On return to the ward, the child is nursed flat. Any restlessness and headache may be alleviated by raising the foot of the bed and administering oxygen. The oxygen assists in absorption of air which has been injected. Temperature may fluctuate considerably following this procedure. Hyperpyrexia is not uncommon, nor is a sudden drop in the temperature leading to shock. It is recommended that the temperature, pulse and respiration be recorded 4-hourly for a 48-hour period following this procedure and more frequently if necessary.

VENTRICULOGRAPHY

The procedure is similar to that of air encephalography except that the air is injected directly into the lateral ventricles.

INFANTS. Where the sutures of the skull have not yet closed, the procedure is the same as for a ventricular puncture (Chapter IX). The scalp may have to be shaved. The requirements are the same as for air encephalography except that a shorter and graduated needle is used. The preparation and care of the child are the same as in air encephalography.

OLDER CHILDREN. The child is prepared as for a general anaesthetic and the scalp is shaved. The procedure is usually carried out by a neuro-surgeon. Bilateral posterior burr holes are made in the skull on either side of the mid-line in the occipital region. A cannula is inserted into the burr hole and passed through the cerebral substance into the posterior horn · of the lateral ventricle.

The care of the child is the same as for air encephalography with additional observations relating to the care of a surgical patient following an intracranial operation; e.g., cerebral irritation, levels of consciousness, signs of infection. Temperature, pulse and respiratory rate should be recorded hourly for the first eight hours and the interval gradually increased to four-hourly by the end of 48 hours.

EXCRETION PYELOGRAM

REASON. This investigation is undertaken when some abnormality of the urinary tract is suspected and to demonstrate the efficiency of renal function.

PRINCIPLE. The opaque medium is normally given intravenously and will be excreted by a functioning kidney a short time afterwards. A series of X-rays taken at the appropriate time will show any deformity of the renal tract from the kidney to the urethra either in outline or in excretion (Fig. 70).

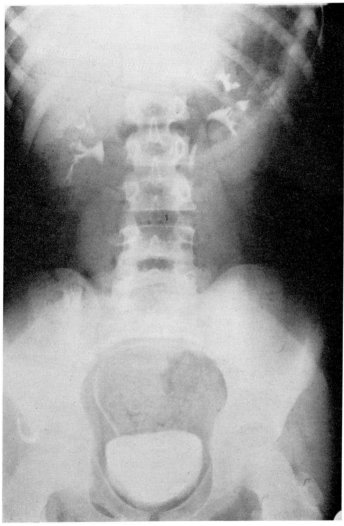

FIG. 70
Intravenous pyelogram showing normal renal tract

REQUIREMENTS:

Sterile equipment :
1. Cleansing swab.
2. 20 ml. syringe and needles No. 12 or 2.
3. Large bore withdrawing needle.

Additional equipment :
4. Warmed ampoule of opaque medium and file.
5. Adrenaline or an antihistamine drug with syringe and needle available to counteract any iodine sensitivity reaction.
6. Receptacle for disposable items.

PREPARATION OF THE CHILD. Ordinary diet is given and bowel action encouraged. If necessary, a suppository may be given the evening before. On the morning of the examination, if the child is well enough, he should be allowed up to run about thus helping the bowel to be rid of gases. Fluids are withheld for six hours prior to the injection but dry food may be given. The child is asked to pass urine before the injection is given. A straight X-ray of the abdomen is taken to exclude renal calculi. The child, if old enough, should be given an adequate explanation of what is going to happen. The injection is usually given into the median basilic vein by the doctor. In small infants a scalp vein may be used, or if a suitable vein is not available, the medium may be given subcutaneously and dispersal aided by hyaluronidase. To test for iodine sensitivity, a test dose of 1 ml. of the substance is injected into a vein. A period of a half minute should elapse and if no reaction occurs, the full amount of the medium can be injected.

Subsequent to the first film after injection, the child is given an aerated drink or the infant, a feed. This demonstrates the left kidney behind the gas bubble formed in the stomach.

SUBCUTANEOUS PYELOGRAM
REQUIREMENTS:

Sterile equipment :
1. Cleansing swab.
2. 20 ml. syringe and needles No. 12.
3. Large bore withdrawing needle.
4. Normal saline temperature 37·8°C or 100°F.

Additional equipment :

5. Warmed ampoule opaque medium and file.
6. Ampoule of hyaluronidase 1,500 units.
7. Water repellent sheet.
8. Receptacle for disposable items.

METHOD. The medium may be diluted with equal parts of normal saline with hyaluronidase added. The dilution of the medium is dependent on the strength and type used. The injection is given into the lateral aspect of the thigh and the infant is transferred to the X-ray department. When giving these drugs intravenously or subcutaneously, it is important to watch for drug idiosyncrasy. Should reactions such as flushing, urticaria, nausea or vomiting occur, the doctor must be notified immediately.

RETROGRADE PYELOGRAPHY

REASON. If kidney function is impaired, intravenous pyelography may fail to give adequate information, and cystoscopy with retrograde pyelography can be performed.

PRINCIPLE. This procedure is carried out under general anaesthesia and a cystoscope is passed into the bladder. Through this instrument, the interior of the bladder is observed and the site of the ureters located. Ureteric catheters are passed through the cystoscope into the bladder and up each ureter to the right and left kidneys. Thus a specimen of urine from the bladder and from each kidney can be obtained. An opaque medium, amount according to age, is injected into each catheter and X-rays are taken.

PREPARATION AND CARE OF THE CHILD. The same preparation is necessary as for excretion pyelogram, with the additional preparation for general anaesthesia. It is not necessary to ensure that the child passes urine prior to the examination, as specimens of urine are to be collected.

Pain and discomfort may follow this examination due to slight trauma of the urethra especially in the male child. There may be haematuria during the first twenty-four hours after the examination and the nurse must ensure that the child is voiding adequate amounts of urine and is not suffering retention because he is afraid to pass urine.

VOIDING CYSTOGRAM

This is a screening procedure to demonstrate the presence of urethral valves and vesico-ureteric reflux.

The bladder is filled with an opaque medium and X-rays are taken when the bladder reaches its capacity. Further X-rays are taken during and on completion of voiding.

REQUIREMENTS. As for catheterisation (Chapter XIV) and additional items:

Sterile equipment :

1. 20 ml. syringe.
2. Jug and large receiver.
3. Spigot or spring clip.
4. Warmed $\frac{1}{2}$ strength normal saline to dilute the opaque medium.

Additional equipment :

5. Opaque medium and file.
6. Adhesive tape to fix to catheter.

PREPARATION OF THE CHILD. A bowel action should be encouraged, or a suppository given the night before the examination. There is no specific preparation on the day other than ensuring that the child understands what is being done and that a nurse he knows remains with him throughout the procedure.

BRONCHOGRAPHY

This is a radiological examination of the lung and is carried out when bronchiectasis is suspected.

PRINCIPLES AND METHOD INVOLVED. This examination is carried out under a general anaesthetic. An iodine-containing contrast medium is injected through an endotracheal tube, under screening control, into the trachea or selected bronchus, and serial X-ray films are then taken to demonstrate the state of the bronchial tree.

Alternatively a fine catheter which fits the syringe and with the tip cut, is attached to the nozzle of the syringe. The catheter is passed via an endotracheal tube. The advantage of the latter procedure is that the medium can be sucked out immediately after the examination is completed.

REQUIREMENTS. Equipment will be required for administering a general anaesthetic. Suction apparatus and resuscitation equipment must all be immediately available (Chapter XX).

SPECIFIC REQUIREMENTS:

1. Swabs.
2. 10 ml. syringe and wide bore withdrawing needles.
3. Catheter No. 9 F.G. or 4 E.G.

Additional equipment :

4. Warmed ampoule of opaque medium and file.
5. Water repellent sheet.
6. Receptacle for disposable items.
7. Receptacle for salvage.

PREPARATION OF THE CHILD. A simple sensitivity test is normally carried out prior to examination to determine any iodine reaction. The day of examination, the child is prepared for a general anaesthetic and suitable explanation is given to the older child. Postural drainage is carried out prior to premedication being given. This is in an attempt to empty the bronchial tubes of as much pus or mucus as possible.

CARE OF THE CHILD. During the immediate post-anaesthetic period, the child requires very close attention. He is nursed in the head low position to facilitate the drainage of any pus or contrast medium, which may contaminate healthy lung tissue. These substances cause an additional hazard in the maintenance of a clear airway and suction with suitable ends must be at the bedside until consciousness has fully returned. The physiotherapist will give treatment at the end of the examination. As soon as the child is fit, postural drainage is repeated and the normal position in bed is resumed thereafter.

CARDIAC CATHETERISATION

Cardiac catheterisation is performed to aid or confirm diagnosis of lesions of the heart and the greater vessels. The pressures within the atrium, ventricles, and pulmonary vessels can be determined. An abnormally high pressure in a ventricle or atria indicates an obstruction to the flow out of that chamber; e.g., pulmonary stenosis. The oxygen content of the blood withdrawn from the various chambers can also be assessed. An unusual oxygen concentration suggests holes in atrial or ventricular septa which permits an abnormal mixture of venous and arterial blood.

PREPARATION OF THE CHILD. A simple explanation should be given to an older child. The nurse from the ward should accompany him and stay with him in the cardiology department. Sedation is given the night previous to the examination and one hour prior to the examination. The child is prepared for a general anaesthetic in case the sedation is not effective. He should be dressed in a theatre gown which is split at the back and tied with tapes. No buttons or pins must be present.

Small infants are dressed in a gamgee jacket and the legs are splinted. The hands are tied with tube-gauze. This allows for change of position for angiocardiography. The child is then covered with a cellular blanket to keep him warm.

When the saphenous vein is being used in babies and small children, it is important to avoid contamination of the wound and catheter by urine and faeces. A Chiron bag is therefore placed in position to collect any urine or faeces passed.

REQUIREMENTS:
1. Sterile pack containing:
   5 dressing towels.
   1 hernia towel (aperature towel).
   1 gown.
   1 hand towel.
   1 pr. gloves.

A large trolley will be necessary with sterile equipment on upper shelf:
2. Tray containing:
   2 ml. syringe for local anaesthetic.
   5 ml. glass syringe.
   3 needles No. 1 and 2.
   2 needles No. 17.
   2 scalpel blades No. 15.
   Length of Portex tubing.
   Plain catgut 2/0.
   Black silk 2/0 with a straight needle.
3. Instruments for venesection:
   1 Double hooked retractor.
   1 Aneurism needle.
   1 Bard-Parker handle No. 3.

1 pr. dissecting forceps.
1 iridectomy forceps.
1 pr. stitch scissors.
1 pr. Mosquito scissors.
2 prs. curved Mosquito forceps.
2 prs. straight Mosquito forceps.
4 towel clips.
   Container with cuvette in sterile water.
4. 3 containers with: Two-way stopcocks.
                      Heller valves.
                      No. 20 needles with little corks.
5. 1 pkt. with Diefenbacher forceps.
6. 3 bowls containing: hexachlorophane 0·5 per cent.
                       5 per cent dextrose in 4/N saline.
                       Empty one for contaminated blood.
7. Packet of swabs.
8. 1 No. 9 F.G. umbilical catheter.
9. Sterile stainless steel syringes 10 ml., 25 ml., 50 ml.

Lower shelf :

1. Small padded splint.
2. 2-inch Elastoplast.
3. Sterile handling forceps.
4. Tube gauze (small size).
5. Chiron bags (small size).
6. Sleek.
7. Scissors.
8. 2 per cent Xylocaine.
9. Heparin 5,000 units per ml.
10. 2 bottles 5 per cent dextrose in 4/N saline.
11. 1 box containing sterile cardiac catheters.
12. Paediatric intravenous giving set.
13. Writing pad and pen.
14. Gamgee jacket for baby.
15. Hot water bottles or heated mattress.
16. Contrast medium.
17. Receptacle for disposable equipment.
18. Receptacle for instruments.
19. Receptacle for syringes.
20. Resuscitation trolley (Chapter XX).

TECHNIQUE. The child lies supine on the X-ray table, which has a 9 in. image intensifier, television camera and a 16 mm. cine camera. Electrodes are placed on the limbs and are connected to an electrocardiographic oscilloscope and a direct writing recorder. The activity of the heart can then be ascertained by the transmission to these machines of the electrical impulses of the heart via the electrodes. The right leg or left arm is then splinted and a

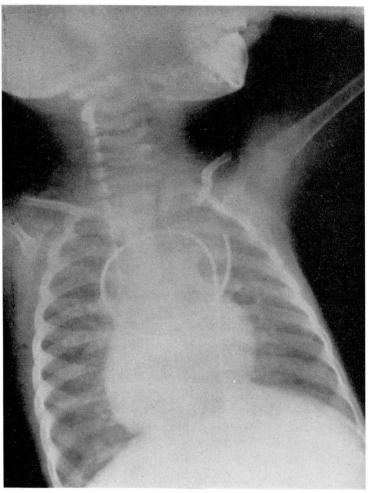

FIG. 71
Cardiac catheterisation

local anaesthetic given in preparation for a venesection. The radio opaque catheter, which is usually 80-100 cm. long, is introduced, under X-ray and television control, into the right saphenous or femoral vein, along the inferior vena cava or, if the left basilic vein is used, along the superior vena cava into the right atrium, right ventricle and then into the pulmonary artery (Fig. 71). With the tip of the catheter at various sites in each chamber and vessel, the other end is connected via the cuvette of a direct reading oximeter and a catheter (umbilical type) to a Statham gauge electro-manometer which measures the pressure wave in that position. The Statham gauge in turn is connected to a direct writing recorder which makes a permanent record. It is also connected to an oscilloscope where the pressure recording can be seen by the cardiologist as he manipulates the catheter.

At each site a specimen of blood is drawn via a 5 ml. glass syringe through the catheter into the cuvette, which rests on a magnetic stirrer over which a photoelectric cell is passed. Immediately the oxygen saturation of the blood at this site has been recorded, the blood specimen in the syringe is returned to the child via the cardiac catheter. A record is kept of the oxygen figures and the site from which these were obtained.

Throughout the catheterisation the catheter is kept patent by an intravenous infusion of 2 bottles of 5 per cent dextrose in $\frac{1}{4}$ strength physiological saline with 5,000 units Heparin added. A careful check is kept on the amount of fluid the child receives during the procedure. One of the bottles is used to wash out the cuvette after the blood specimen used for oximetry has been returned to the child, and is directed through the cuvette to be discarded via a rubber tube to a basin standing on the floor.

At the completion of the catheterisation and angiocardiography, the amount of fluid received and the time exposed to radiation are recorded.

Angiocardiography

This is an X-ray study of the heart and is useful in the diagnosis of cardiac anomalies. The open-ended catheter used for the catheterisation is withdrawn, and a special catheter with six perforations close to the tip is inserted. This type of catheter eliminates the risk of damaging the endocardium when injecting the contrast medium under high pressure and prevents catheter recoil.

TECHNIQUE. A test injection of the contrast medium is given during catheterisation. The catheter tip is introduced into that part of the heart or vessel where a defect is suspected and where most information will be obtained.

A stainless steel syringe is filled with the contrast medium and all air is expelled. The amount of contrast medium used depends on the weight of the child. The pressure of the injection is regulated by a pneumatic pump and depends on the site of the catheter and the nature of the defect. The syringe is placed in a metal cradle and is attached to the cardiac catheter and to the pneumatic pump. The cine camera records the passage of the fluid through the heart chambers and the great vessels.

Aortography

This is performed in much the same way as angiography; the contrast medium is injected under pressure into the ascending aorta, the catheter having been advanced into the aorta via the femoral or brachial artery.

AFTER CARE. When the examinations are completed, the child is returned to the ward and kept warm. Shock may sometimes occur, and it is therefore important to observe the child frequently, disturbing him as little as possible for the first four hours. The pulse rate should be recorded $\frac{1}{2}$ hourly or more frequently, as necessary. Any napkin changes or other nursing care should be carried out gently.

BIBLIOGRAPHY

Ministry of Health (1966). *Code of Practice for the Protection of Persons against Ionising Radiations arising from Medical and Dental Use.* London: H.M.S.O.
Munro, J. M. (1967). *Pre-Nursing Course in Science*, 2nd ed., chap. 12. Edinburgh: Livingstone.
Watts, J. (1963). Cardiac catheterisation. *Nurs. Mirror*, **117**, 3060.

CHAPTER XVII

METABOLIC TESTS AND OTHERS

Sweat test; duodenal intubation; jejunal biopsy; abdominal paracentesis; peritoneal dialysis; fat balance; liver biopsy; Guthrie's test; urine tests.

SWEAT TEST (THERMAL)

REASON AND PRINCIPLE INVOLVED. In this procedure, the aim is to encourage the excretion of sweat, so that the contents of the sweat may be analysed. It is an important aid to diagnosis in the condition of fibrocystic disease of the pancreas, where the concentration of chlorides in sweat is increased.

There are various methods of carrying out this test and mention will be made of two which are generally used. Stimulation of sweat can be achieved in two ways; firstly, by the application of general heat; and, secondly, by the local stimulation of the sweat glands in a limited area by the use of chemicals. The first method is largely being superseded by the second one as it avoids the discomfort and danger inherent in severe generalised sweating.

REQUIREMENTS:

1. Dissecting forceps.
2. Swabs.
3. 2 gallipots for skin cleansing lotion and methylated ether.
4. Square piece of jaconet slightly larger than the swab.
5. 1 in. adhesive strapping.
6. 1 pr. scissors.
7. Jar with lid containing a weighed swab.
8. Receptacle for used swabs.
9. 4 covered hot water bottles.
10. 4 blankets.
11. Plastic bag.
12. Change of clothing.
13. Bathing equipment.

PREPARATION AND CARE OF THE CHILD. It is important to remember that excessive sweating will lead to loss of water and chlorides, so that the child may become dehydrated, a condition which leads to respiratory distress and cyanosis. It is therefore necessary to prepare drinks containing salt; e.g., orange juice in $\frac{1}{2}$ strength normal saline, or for infants $\frac{1}{4}$ or $\frac{1}{2}$ strength normal saline. This can be given during and after the test. While the test is in progress, constant supervision is necessary. The room must be warm and the bed prepared by placing well covered hot water bottles in it, or, if available, by using a well protected electric blanket. The child is undressed and placed inside the plastic bag enclosing the whole body except the head. Before closing the bag, the area between the two scapulae is washed with methylated ether to remove any skin oils and inorganic salts. A swab, which has been weighed previously and is completely dry, is placed on the cleaned area with a pair of forceps. This swab is covered with a piece of jaconet slightly bigger than the swab and is held in position by adhesive tape. The bag is then closed at the neck and the child covered by blankets. Sweating should be profuse and beads of sweat on the forehead and neck will indicate when to remove the child from the sweat bag. During this time the child must be watched carefully for any signs of respiratory distress, cyanosis or dehydration. Whenever any of these signs appear, doctor must be notified and the test abandoned. Oxygen should be administered and saline drinks given.

When sweating is profuse, the swab is removed with a pair of forceps, placed into the jar provided, and sent to the biochemistry department for analysis.

Meanwhile the child is given a drink and a bath is prepared and given. Cooling of the child must be avoided, therefore bathing and dressing should take place in a warm room and the clothing should be warmed.

Instead of using the plastic bag, blankets only may be used. The child is wrapped in the blankets overnight and the test is discontinued in the morning. The care of the child is the same as in the method described above.

SWEAT TEST BY IONTOPHORESIS

This method causes much less distress to the child, but requires extremely accurate calculation, as the quantity of sweat obtained is so minute. A chemical such as Pilocarpine is used; the ionised drug is transported to the sweat glands under the influence of an electric field. No special preparation of the child is required, and no special restrictions need to be placed on the child immediately before or after the procedure. The older child should be given a simple explanation to allay his fears and gain his co-operation

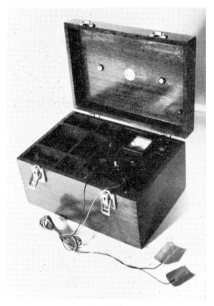

FIG. 72
Sweat test box

REQUIREMENTS:

1. Sweat test box (Fig. 72).
2. Specially weighed container and filter paper from the laboratory (to absorb the sweat).
3. Solution of Pilocarpine nitrate 0·2 per cent in distilled water (increases sweating).
4. Solution of Magnesium sulphate 10 per cent.
5. Lint and gauze swabs.
6. Square of polythene or oiled silk about 6 in. square.
7. Distilled or deionised water and ether for skin cleansing.
8. Waterproof adhesive.
9. 3 prs. dissecting forceps and scissors.

10. 3 small gallipots for solutions which must be free from electrolyte contaminations.

PREPARATION OF EQUIPMENT.

1. Two pads, each of 5 thicknesses of lint, are made of slightly larger size than the electrode plates.
2. Polythene or oiled silk is cut to about 6 in. square, large enough to cover the filter paper completely with about 1 in. overlap, or sufficiently large to cover the area between the scapulae.
3. Strips of waterproof adhesive are prepared, to seal off completely the edges of the waterproof sheet. These are applied after the filter paper and polythene sheet are in position on the skin.

METHOD. Areas of the skin on which the electrodes are to be placed are cleaned to remove old sebaceous secretion and sweat. Ether is used, followed by distilled or deionised water and the areas are then dried.

One pad of lint is moistened with magnesium sulphate solution and placed on the child's thigh. The electrode plate is placed on top and, using waterproof adhesive, the assembly is strapped to the thigh sufficiently firmly to make good contact. This electrode is connected to the negative lead. The magnesium sulphate solution provides the electrolyte necessary for the conduction of the electric current.

The second pad is moistened with the Pilocarpine solution and placed on a suitable area of the thorax where the filter paper can later be applied flat; e.g., the area between the scapulae. The electrode plate and strapping is applied as before and connection is made to the positive lead.

Great care must be taken to ensure that no part of the electrode plate or any bare lead touches the skin or a burn may be produced when current is passed.

When both leads are securely in position, the doctor adjusts the current gradually to 4-5 milliamps and leaves it at this level for 5 minutes. The child may feel a slight tingling sensation.

The electrodes and pads are then removed. A reddened area will be seen under the Pilocarpine electrode. The area and some distance around is washed with distilled or deionised water to remove Pilocarpine and sweat already on the skin. The area is then dried completely, making sure that no threads or paper fluff remain which might adhere to the filter paper.

The filter paper is removed from the container with clean forceps and applied to the reddened area. The waterproof sheet is placed on top and is sealed off with waterproof adhesive to give an airtight seal. A cross of adhesive in the middle will help to hold the paper in better contact with the skin. The filter paper is left in place for 40-60 minutes, and it is then carefully removed with clean forceps. Great care must be taken to ensure that the filter paper is intact and no part is broken off. It is placed at once in the bottle or container which must be closed and sent to the laboratory as soon as possible for analysis.

The skin areas used are then carefully cleaned and any adhesive removed.

PRECAUTIONS WHEN PERFORMING THE TEST. The dangers of burning have already been mentioned and great care must be taken in preventing this. Contamination with sodium must be avoided, as this would affect the analysis. Soap and detergents must be rigorously excluded from any part in the test. The filter paper and anything which touches it must be handled with forceps only, to avoid risk of contamination from the operator's hands. No material used in the test should be laid on surfaces which might be contaminated with sodium salts. No saline solution must be used at any stage.

Evaporation must be avoided by ensuring an airtight seal between skin and waterproof covering, by rapid transfer of the damp paper to the bottle, and by airtight closure of the bottle.

Since the complete bottle and filter paper have been weighed, no label should be applied to it, but the number of the bottle is used for identification on the request form. Care must also be taken to avoid damage which might alter the weight of the bottle.

DUODENAL INTUBATION

REASON. Duodenal fluid is obtained by passing a duodenal tube into the duodenum. Examination of the fluids yields valuable information concerning the character of the fluid and its enzyme content. The fluid is normally clear and watery, it may be colourless or of varying shades of yellow, depending on its bile content. It is alkaline in reaction containing the enzymes trypsin, amylase, and lipase. This test is carried out as an aid to the diagnosis of fibrocystic disease of the pancreas. In this disease mucosis and fibrosis of the glandular tissue occurs, leading to deficiency or absence of pancreatic enzymes in the duodenal juice. For practical purposes the fluid need only be tested for the presence of trypsin. A very low amount or absence of trypsin is indicative of the disease.

REQUIREMENTS:

1. Duodenal or Ryles tubes (new or fairly stiff) size No. 11 F.G. or No. 6 E.G.
2. 20 ml. syringe.
3. Container for rejected fluid.
4. Stand with 6-10 test tubes.
5. Bowl containing ice to keep the specimen cool.
6. Swabs.
7. Container with normal saline.
8. Red litmus paper.
9. Safety pin and spigot.
10. Adhesive tape.
11. Vomit bowl (for older child).

PREPARATION AND CARE OF THE CHILD. When the child is old enough a simple explanation should be given and his co-operation obtained. The older child is prepared by giving nothing by mouth from 10 p.m. The infant is usually given a feed at 6 a.m. but the 10 a.m. feed is omitted.

PREPARATION OF THE OLDER CHILD. The child lies in the right lateral position as this appears to aid the tube to gravitate into the duodenum. Until the tube is passed, the hands may have to be restrained. A nurse should stay with the child and amuse him during the procedure which may take some considerable time.

PREPARATION OF THE INFANT. The infant is sedated prior to this procedure. He is wrapped in a cotton blanket and the arms are restrained. Like the older child, he lies in the right lateral position.

The tube is then passed gently either through the mouth or nose into the stomach and finally directed towards the pyloric orifice. The tube must be secured to the face to prevent it being sucked into the intestines. In some units the child may be X-rayed to ascertain the position of the tube. At intervals of 10-15 minutes, the syringe is attached and fluid aspirated until bile-stained fluid is obtained. When clear yellow fluid has been obtained it should be tested with litmus paper, and, if alkaline in reaction, it is placed into the bowl containing the ice and taken to the biochemistry department. It is wise to ascertain the relative value of the fluid first before removing the tube. When the tube is removed, the child is made comfortable and a feed or meal is given.

Alternatively, the tube may be passed in the X-ray department when a Levin's opaque catheter is used and screening will ascertain that the catheter is actually in the duodenum.

JEJUNAL BIOPSY

REASON. This is a reliable test carried out to diagnose coeliac disease. In this disease there appears to be an enzyme defect in the cells of the intestinal mucosa which results in the defective splitting of the glutamine-containing peptides of gliadin into amino-acids. Children affected by this disease are unable to metabolise gluten found in wheat and rye flour. Various other defects in absorption may become apparent.

The purpose of this biopsy is to obtain a specimen from the duodenum or jejunum. This will show flat mucosa which is devoid of normal villi.

REQUIREMENTS:

1. As for passing a naso-gastric tube with the addition of a special Crosby catheter.
2. Water repellent sheet.
3. Swabs.
4. Vomit bowl.
5. Adhesive tape.
6. Scissors.
7. Restraining sleeves.
8. Jar for specimen.

PREPARATION OF THE CHILD. If the child is old enough, a simple explanation should be given. No food or drink is given from 12 midnight. Sedation is given to the child. He is placed in the right lateral position with both hands restrained to the right side of the cot. This is to assist the tube to gravitate into the duodenum.

CARE OF THE CHILD DURING THE PROCEDURE. The catheter is passed by the doctor. The mother or a nurse remains with the child and ensures that he remains in the same position. Restlessness must be prevented and care taken that the tube is not pulled out. Three hours later the child is taken to the X-ray department and the position of the capsule is determined by X-ray screening. If the position is satisfactory, the doctor takes a specimen and removes the tube.

AFTER CARE OF THE CHILD. The child is made comfortable and nursed in bed for the rest of the day. Fluids only are given on the day of the test. This procedure carries a small risk of haemorrhage or perforation. It is therefore essential to observe the child carefully. The pulse rate is recorded hourly for the first four hours. Any vomit must be kept for inspection and the presence of blood reported immediately. Should the child complain of any pain, this must be reported without delay. Any stools passed should be tested for faecal occult blood.

ABDOMINAL PARACENTESIS

REASON. This is performed to withdraw serous fluid from the peritoneal cavity. Under normal conditions this fluid is produced by the peritoneum and functions as a lubricant to the abdominal viscera. Gross increase of fluid occurs in certain pathological conditions and causes the abdomen to become distended. This is called abdominal ascites and will lead to respiratory embarrassment. It is usually the symptom of a serious disease. Some of the causes in children may be nephrotic syndrome, cardiac failure, or Banti's syndrome.

REQUIREMENTS:

Sterile equipment :
1. Swabs.
2. Cleansing lotions.
3. Southey's trocar and cannula with fine rubber tubing.
4. 1 ml. syringe and No. 17 needles.
5. Scalpel and blade.
6. Dissecting forceps.
7. Skin suture needle and silk.

Additional equipment :
8. Water repellent sheet.
9. Clip to regulate the flow.

10. Uribag.
11. Planocaine 1 per cent.
12. Abdominal binder, safety pins and adhesive tape.
13. Receptacle for disposable items.
14. Receptacle for salvage.

PREPARATION OF THE CHILD. Sedation is usually given to allay
fear and restlessness. The child is kept in bed supported by two
pillows. The bladder must be emptied immediately before the
paracentesis is done. Catheterisation is performed, if necessary,
because of the danger of puncturing a distended bladder. A
cradle is required to prevent pressure of bedclothes on the abdomen. The child is dressed in warm light clothing and a water
repellent sheet is placed under the child. An abdominal binder
is placed in position so that it can be applied as soon as the cannula is inserted.

METHOD. The procedure is carried out by the doctor under local
anaesthesia. A Southey's trocar and cannula is introduced and
fine rubber tubing is attached, which should be long enough to
reach into the collecting uribag. Where difficulty is experienced
in introducing the trocar and cannula, a small incision may be
made with a scalpel. In this case the doctor may wish to insert a
skin suture when the procedure is completed. The cannula is
held in position with a dressing and adhesive tape.

CARE DURING DRAINAGE. The drainage is often continued for
twenty-four hours and the amount of fluid drained may be several
litres. This may lead to weakness and faintness. During the
treatment the child must be watched carefully. Firm pressure is
maintained on the abdomen by means of the abdominal binder,
which must be adjusted according to the decrease of abdominal
distension. The level in the collecting bag is noted and the fluid
should be measured and charted before it is emptied. The
nutritional needs of the child must be catered for. If repeated
paracentesis is necessary, there is a considerable loss of body
proteins and therefore the diet should be rich in protein. Extra
carbohydrate and full vitamin supplement are required where liver
damage impairs glycogen storage and the production of vitamin K.
When fat digestion is impaired due to inadequate production of
bile, only a minimum of fatty food should be given.

AFTER CARE. When the drainage is completed, the cannula is

withdrawn and the puncture is dressed with a dry, sterile swab. The binder is then reapplied and the child is made comfortable.

PERITONEAL DIALYSIS

PRINCIPLES INVOLVED. Dialysis is the process whereby crystalloids; i.e., small molecules such as sodium chloride, and some colloids; i.e., large molecules such as sugar in a solution are separated. This is made possible by the passage of these substances through a semi-permeable membrane by *diffusion*. This membrane permits the transfer of water molecules and crystalloids but not larger molecules. For example; the separation of water and sugar; water will pass into the sugar solution but sugar will not pass out. The sugar solution becomes diluted and increases in volume. The sugar molecules act as though they are attracting water molecules across the membrane. The process of transference of water across a membrane is called *osmosis* and the pressure created by the increased volume is *osmotic pressure*. The processes of dialysis and osmosis play a vital part in the interchange of fluid between the blood and the fluid of the tissues.

There are many such membranes in the body. One example is the peritoneum which lines the abdominal and pelvic cavities. Functions of this membrane include: protection against bacteria, reduction of friction, secretion of serous fluid, and the ability to allow the passage of substances through the membrane. It is the latter function of which use is made in the procedure of peritoneal dialysis.

REASON. This is a process by which dangerous end products of protein metabolism, or poisonous substances, can be removed from the body. This method can be used in renal failure where the aim is to remove excessive urea from the blood or where barbiturate or salicylate poisoning has occurred. It is carried out by passing a salt and sugar solution or dextrose into the peritoneal cavity. Use is made of the lining of the patient's own abdominal cavity as the dialysing membrane. The solution attracts to itself, through the peritoneal lining, the nitrogenous products or other substances which are not being excreted by the patient's kidneys. Urea and other substances in the blood diffuse through the peritoneal lining into the dialysing solution which is then removed by syphonage. Where oedema is present in association with renal failure or acute congestive cardiac failure, a hypertonic solution of 7 per cent

Dextrose will remove the excess fluid by increasing the 'osmotic pull'.

REQUIREMENTS:

Sterile equipment :
1. Dianeal administration set.
2. Peritoneal dialysis catheter.
3. 10 ml. syringe and No. 1 needles.
   2 ml. syringe and No. 17 needles.
4. Containers for skin cleansing lotions.
5. Cotton wool balls.
6. Swabs.
7. Scalpel blade and handle.
   2 prs. dissecting forceps.
   1 pr. artery forceps.

Additional equipment :
8. Sterile water.
9. Heparin 5,000 I.U.
10. Achromycin I.V. 250 mg.
11. Ampoules of pot. chloride.
    Ampoules of calcium chloride.
    Ampoules of sod. bicarbonate.
    2 vials 50 ml. Mannitol.
    5 vials 250 mg. Aldomet.
12. Files.
13. Fluid chart.
14. Adhesive tape.
15. Dialysing fluid—7 per cent dextrose; 1·5 per cent dextrose —all bottles must be accurately numbered.
16. Lotion thermometer.
17. Container to heat the dialysing fluid.
18. Containers for laboratory specimens.
19. Many-tailed binder and safety pins or Netalast.
20. Large container for returned fluid.
21. Receptacle for disposable items.
22. Receptacle for salvage.
23. Receptacle for used apparatus.

PREPARATION OF THE CHILD. A simple explanation should be given to the child if he is old enough. It may be necessary to restrain his arms to prevent him from touching the tubing. Usually a local anaesthetic is given, but sedation may also be necessary to allay fear and restlessness. The procedure is carried out in the operating theatre. Before being taken to the operating theatre the child is asked to void urine but if he is unconscious or unable to do so, he is catheterised. An indwelling catheter may be left in position. This is important because of the danger of puncturing a distended bladder. The child is dressed in warm light clothing and a water repellent sheet is placed under him.

METHOD. An incision is made in the mid-line of the abdomen. A special peritoneal catheter is introduced which is held in position with a swab and adhesive tape. The special set is then attached to the catheter and the vacolitre. The fluid to be used is heated by immersing the vacolitre in a water bath at 40°C (104°F). Heparin is added to the fluid to prevent fibrin formation.

The amount of fluid allowed to run into the peritoneum varies with the age of the child. For a 7-year-old and upwards it may be 500 ml., with less fluid for the younger child. The warmed fluid is allowed to run in for 20-30 minutes, and remains in the peritoneal cavity for 30 minutes. During this time dialysis occurs. The vacolitres are then lowered and placed below the level of the insertion of the catheter, beside the bed, and the fluid is allowed to syphon back over a period of 20 minutes. A specimen of the returned fluid is sent for estimation and analysis to the biochemistry department. If the flow of fluid stops or slows down, the catheter tip may be moved slightly.

CARE OF THE CHILD. The child is placed on his back with one pillow under his head. His temperature is taken and recorded hourly; children become readily chilled due to loss of fluid and this could lead to shock and a fall in blood pressure. The room should be warm but overheating of the child should be avoided. The first fluid syphoned back may be bloodstained. Pain and discomfort may also be present due to the increased amount of fluid in the peritoneal cavity. An abdominal binder may be applied to support the emptying abdomen.

Once the procedure is completed, the cannula is removed and the wound dressed. A dumbbell adhesive dressing may be used to seal the wound; alternatively, sutures may be required and a dressing applied. If stitches are inserted, they are removed on the 7th or 8th day.

FAT BALANCE

REASON. To determine the fat content in faeces, to aid or confirm the diagnosis of coeliac disease, congenital fibrocystic disease of the pancreas, and infantile steatorrhoea.

Normal faecal fat varies with different age-levels and the total fat from two to six months is 0·3-1·3 grammes per day. From six months to six years 0·33-1·8 grammes per day. A daily output in excess of 4 grammes in a child indicates steatorrhoea.

METHOD.

1. The child is given a diet containing a known amount of fat according to his weight. The diet is given for two days to determine how the child will manage the diet. It consists of fatless foods, plus the required amount of known fat in milk. This is usually divided into milk to be taken at ward level as drinks and milk puddings. Rejected food is returned to the diet kitchen for estimation. The only foods allowed to be given to the child from the ward are orange juice and water. The test should be explained to the parents and their co-operation sought so that no other food is given to the child. It is also advisable to detail a nurse per shift of duty to care for the child, and take full responsibility in ensuring that the diet is given to the child, and to collect the stools which are passed.

2. The child is given a carmine marker (A). This consists of one capsule, which is given at the end of the *second* day of the diet, i.e. 10 p.m.

3. The diet is given for *five* days.

4. At the end of the fifth day at 10 p.m. a carmine marker (B) is given to the child.

5. The diet is continued for one more day.

Stool Collection

1. The first *pink* stool containing marker (A) is *discarded*. It is recorded and noted as the commencement of the collection.

2. All stools passed per 24 hours (10 p.m.-10 p.m.) are put in one container and marked with the name of the child, date and day of balance.

3. The first *pink* stool containing marker (B) is the last stool to be collected.

4. Polythene sheets can be used inside the potty or bedpan to collect the stools. In the case of infants, the napkin may be lined with a polythene sheet which should be changed frequently to prevent sore buttocks. In some units, the infant is sat on a special chair and the stools are collected in the pan placed underneath the chair (Fig. 54).

While the test is in progress, a fluid balance chart is maintained. Any vomitus is collected and sent to the biochemistry laboratory at the same time as the stools. The container must be labelled containing the child's name, date and time the vomiting occurred. If it is not possible to save the vomitus, an accurate report must be sent to the laboratory.

At the completion of the fat balance test, the dietician brings the chart containing the total daily fat intake, while the chart containing the total daily output is obtained from the biochemistry department. From this, the total daily and overall absorption is calculated. Absorption of fat should be 90-96 per cent of the intake.

EXAMINATION FOR TRYPTIC ACTIVITY

This examination is carried out when a child presents a history of loose stools. Specimens of faeces are sent to the biochemical department. Stools are analysed for the presence of trypsin. Trypsin is a protealytic enzyme which is one of the pancreatic enzymes. In fibrocystic disease of the pancreas the enzymes cannot reach the digestive tract. The test is usually done only for trypsin and in these cases the result may show diminished or absent tryptic activity.

GUTHRIE'S TEST

REASON. This is a screening test to detect cases of phenyl-ketonuria in very early infancy. The test is carried out by the sixth day of life when feeding is established, and the serum level of phenylalanine may be high.

REQUIREMENTS:

1. Heel stab needle.
2. Swabs.

3. Mediswab or cleansing lotion; e.g., isopropyl alcohol.
4. Elastoplast dressing.
5. Guthrie's test card.
6. Receptacle for disposable items.

METHOD. The skin is cleansed with isopropyl alcohol. This liquid dries quickly thereby decreasing the possibility of contamination which would invalidate the test. The heel is stabbed and a drop of blood is placed on each of the four rings on the special test card. The punctured area on the heel is cleaned and light pressure is applied to stop bleeding with an Elastoplast dressing. The test card is then completed in pencil and sent to the biochemistry laboratory.

LIVER BIOPSY

REASON. This procedure is carried out in children suspected of suffering from cirrhosis of the liver or tumours of the liver.

TECHNIQUE. A special liver puncture needle is inserted into the liver, passing between the lower ribs. As the needle passes through the liver tissue, it cuts a long core of tissue which remains in the barrel of the needle. The specimen of liver tissue is placed in formol-saline solution and sent to the pathological laboratory.

REQUIREMENTS:

Sterile equipment :

1. Containers with cleansing lotions.
2. Cotton wool balls.
3. Container with normal saline.
4. 2 Menghini liver biopsy needles with obdurator.
5. 20 ml. glass leur-lock syringe.
6. 2 × 2 ml., 2 × 10 ml., 2 × 2 ml. disposable syringes.
   Disposable needles Nos. 1, 15, 21.
7. Scalpel and blade.
8. 4 dressing towels as drapes.
   1 sterile hand towel.
   Gowns.

Additional equipment :

9. Ethyl chloride spray. ⎱ if required.
10. Lignocaine 1 per cent. ⎰
11. Filter paper.
12. Sterile universal container.
    Sterile universal container with 10 per cent formol-saline.
13. Masks.
14. Resuscitation equipment (Chapter XX).

PREPARATION OF THE CHILD. A simple explanation should be given to the child, if he is old enough. He is prepared as for a general anaesthetic. Premedication may be ordered and should be given at the time stated. The procedure may be carried out while the child is anaesthetised with Sodium Thiopentone administered rectally (see Chapter VIII).

CARE OF THE CHILD. Throughout the procedure and following it, careful observation must be kept on the child's pulse and respiration. Complications such as haemorrhage may arise, particularly if the biopsy is carried out for a tumour of the liver. After the procedure, the child is nursed in the sitting position supported by three pillows. A cradle is inserted to keep the weight of the bedclothes off the abdomen.

URINE TESTING

Urine contains the byproducts of body metabolism with the exception of carbon dioxide.

Examination of the urine may reveal valuable information which can be an important aid to diagnosis. It is essential, therefore, that all tests carried out should be accurately performed. It is unwise to rely on memory when using an unfamiliar chemical test. The smallest error in the amount of reagent can give an erroneous result.

Urine to be tested must be fresh, as changes in its composition occur when it is allowed to stand; e.g., in glycosuria, the type of sugar alters on standing. The alteration will affect the result of the test. It is also important to collect the specimen of urine in a clean receptacle.

General Examination

QUANTITY. The volume of output varies considerably in

different age-groups and is also dependent on the amount of fluid intake as well as the fluid lost from the body by other routes.

POLYURIA, or increased urinary output, occurs in diabetes insipidus and uncontrolled diabetes mellitus.

OLIGURIA, or diminished urinary output, occurs in acute nephritis, and conditions associated with dehydration.

ODOUR. Abnormal odours: (1) the sweet smell of acetone; (2) the fishy smell when there is a cystitis; (3) ammoniacal smell (when urine is allowed to stand, this will develop, due to bacterial decomposition of urea to ammonia); (4) smell of honey found in infants suffering from phenylketonuria.

REACTION. Normally urine is slightly acid and will turn blue litmus paper red.

SEDIMENT. Normally there is no sediment, but when urine is left to stand, a deposit may be seen. Urates form a pale pink curd-like sediment. Phosphates form a white sediment.

SPECIFIC GRAVITY. Normal 1·015 to 1·025. This is recorded by floating a urinometer in urine. The reading is taken at eye level and care must be taken not to have the urinometer touching the sides of the container. The urine should be at room temperature.

Where there is a diminished output, as in a febrile state, the specific gravity is found to be high. When there is an increased output, normally the specific gravity is low. The exception to this is in diabetes mellitus when the high sugar content of the urine makes the specific gravity high.

CHLORIDES

Normally chlorides are present in the urine. Absence denotes a chloride deficiency which may be due to loss through excessive vomiting, or to continuous gastric aspiration.

FANTUS TEST

Purpose: To estimate amount of chloride.

EQUIPMENT. Test tube. Pipette with rubber end. 20 per cent potassium chromate solution. 2·9 per cent silver nitrate solution. Distilled water for rinsing.

METHOD. Rinse the test tube and pipette with distilled water. Place ten drops of urine in the test tube and rinse the pipette again. Add one drop of potassium chromate and rinse the pipette.

Add the silver nitrate drop by drop until a sharp colour change from yellow to reddish brown occurs. Assessment of amount of chlorides is made by counting the number of drops of silver nitrate necessary for the colour change. The number is equivalent to grammes of chloride per litre of urine. The normal is between three and five. The doctor will also require to know the amount of urine passed in twenty-four hours and the specific gravity of the specimen in order to interpret the result.

TESTS FOR PROTEIN

Purpose : Detection of urinary tract disease.

1. Boiling Test

REQUIREMENTS. One test tube. Spirit lamp, or bunsen burner. One pipette with rubber bulb. 10 per cent acetic acid. Filter paper and funnel, if necessary.

METHOD. Filter urine if any cloudiness is present. The top inch of a test tube three-quarters full of urine is boiled over a spirit lamp. The tube should be rotated gently during the process to prevent cracking. After boiling, the urine at the top of the tube is compared with the lower unboiled part. The presence of a cloud denotes either phosphates or protein. Three drops of 10 per cent acetic acid is added and the top portion reboiled. Disappearance of the cloud indicates phosphates; persistence of the cloud indicates protein.

2. Salicylsulphonic Acid Test

REQUIREMENTS. One test tube. One pipette with rubber bulb. 25 per cent solution salicylsulphonic acid. Filter paper and funnel if necessary.

METHOD. Filter the urine if any cloudiness is present. Put approximately 5 ml. urine in a test tube and add five drops of a 25 per cent solution of salicylsulphonic acid. If protein is present, the urine will become cloudy. The heavier the cloud, the more evidence of protein.

3. Albustix

REQUIREMENTS. Albustix reagent strip. Colour chart.

METHOD. Dip test end of strip in the urine and remove immediately. Compare the colour with the colour scale. The end will turn green in the presence of protein.

4. Uristix for protein and glucose

REQUIREMENTS. Uristix reagent strip, colour chart.

METHOD. Dip protein portion in the urine and remove immediately. The end will turn green within 10 seconds in the presence of protein. If the test is for glucose, the glucose portion (nearer the middle) will turn purple within 10 seconds.

5. Esbach's Test

This is a useful test when it is desirable to estimate the quantity of protein in the urine. It may be carried out daily over a period of weeks, gradually decreasing amounts of proteinuria denoting increasing renal efficiency.

REQUIREMENTS. Urinometer, Esbach's albuminometer. Esbach's reagent. Litmus paper. 10 per cent acetic acid if necessary. Collection of urine over a twenty-four hour period.

METHOD. The twenty-four hour collection of urine is well mixed and a sample taken. The specific gravity is recorded and if this is above 1·010 the urine is diluted with water, and the final result is multiplied by the requisite number of times. The urine must be acid; it is therefore tested with litmus paper and, if alkaline, a few drops of 10 per cent acetic acid are added until the reaction changes.

1. Pour the urine into the Esbach's tube until it reaches the letter U.

2. Add Esbach's reagent up to the letter R.

3. Lock the tube and invert gently two or three times to ensure thorough mixing of the contents.

4. Place the tube upright in the stand and leave in a constant temperature for twenty-four hours.

5. The reading is taken at eye level when the depth of the sediment is measured against the scale on the albuminometer. This gives the amount of protein in the urine in parts per thousand, or grammes per litre.

The main constituent of the reagent is picric acid and it is this which precipitates the protein.

P.N.P.—L

TESTS FOR SUGAR

1. Clinistix—Detection of Glucose

REQUIREMENTS. Clinistix. Colour chart.

METHOD. Dip the test end of the Clinistix into the urine and remove. Examine both sides of the stick after one minute for the presence of a blue colour. A positive reaction, which denotes the presence of glucose in the urine, is demonstrated when the stick turns blue within one minute.

2. Uristix for protein and glucose

REQUIREMENTS. Uristix reagent strip. Colour chart.

METHOD. Dip glucose portion in the urine. If glucose is present it will turn purple within 10 seconds. If it is negative and tests are required for sugars other than glucose; e.g., Galactose, Clinitest tablets should be used.

3. Clinitest—Estimation of Urine Sugar

REQUIREMENTS. Clinitest reagent tablets. Pipette with rubber bulb. Test tube. Colour chart.

METHOD. Place five drops of urine into a test tube. Rinse dropper and add ten drops of water. Drop in one Clinitest tablet and watch the reaction. Fifteen seconds after boiling stops, shake the tube gently and compare with the Clinitest colour scale.

Negative Reaction. All shades of blue are negative.

Positive Reaction. Colour change to green, brown, or orange indicates that sugar is present. Should the colour change rapidly through the stages to brown, a reading is taken as over 2 per cent.

4. Benedict's Test

REQUIREMENTS. Benedict's qualitative reagent. Test tube. Bunsen burner, or spirit lamp.

METHOD. Place 5 ml. Benedict's qualitative reagent into a test tube and add eight drops of urine. Boil the mixture vigorously for two minutes.

In the presence of sugar, the colour will change to bluish-green, green, yellow, orange, and finally brick red, depending on the quantity of sugar present.

Substances other than glucose may give a positive reaction to the Clinitest and to Benedict's test. Salicylates give a positive reaction. A positive reaction to Clinistix is positive proof of the presence of glucose.

TESTS FOR KETONE BODIES

Purpose : Forewarning of diabetic coma or acidosis.

1. Acetest

REQUIREMENTS. Acetest tablet. Paper square. Pipette with rubber bulb. Colour chart.

METHOD. Place an Acetest tablet on a clean surface, preferably a piece of white paper. Put one drop of urine on the tablet. Take the reading in thirty seconds and compare the colour of the tablet with the colour scale and record as negative, trace, moderate, or strongly positive. Negative remains white. Positive turns mauve.

This test is the most reliable in the presence of ketone bodies and is not affected by the administration of salicylates.

2. Ketostix. Test for ketones

REQUIREMENTS. Ketostix reagent strips. Colour chart.

METHOD. Urine must be freshly passed and absolutely free from contaminants and clean. Dip test end into the urine and remove immediately. Exactly 15 seconds later compare the test end part with the colour chart. Lavender or purple colour indicates the presence of ketones. The colour block indicates the degree of ketosis present.

3. Rothera's Test

REQUIREMENTS. Ammonium sulphate crystals. 2 per cent sodium nitro-prusside solution, or crystals. Strong ammonia. Test tube. Pipette with rubber bulb.

METHOD. Place half an inch of ammonium sulphate crystals in the test tube and add 5 ml. urine to make a saturated solution. Ten drops of freshly prepared 2 per cent sodium nitro-prusside solution is added and the solution well mixed. Alternatively, two crystals of sodium nitro-prusside are added and the mixture shaken well. Ten drops of strong ammonia are run down the side of the test tube. A purple coloured ring will develop if acetone or diacetic acid is present.

The depth of colour and the speed at which it develops indicate the amount of acetone present. A pinkish colour may develop which is of no significance.

This test is a very sensitive one and may show a positive reaction if the patient has not eaten for several hours.

4. Gerhardt's Test

This test is not always reliable, as it is only positive when fairly large quantities of acetone are present in the urine.

REQUIREMENTS. 10 per cent ferric chloride. Test tube. Pipette with rubber bulb.

METHOD. Put 2 ml. urine into the test tube and add 10 per cent ferric chloride solution drop by drop. The urine becomes cloudy as phosphates are precipitated, and if diacetic acid is present a reddish-brown colour develops.

It is important to know if salicylates in any form; e.g., aspirin, are being taken, as this test will then give a positive reaction.

TEST FOR BLOOD

Purpose : Detection of kidney or urinary tract disease

1. Occultest Reagent Tablets

REQUIREMENTS. Occultest reagent tablets. Pipette with rubber bulb. Filter paper and square.

METHOD. Place one drop of well mixed uncentrifuged urine on the centre of the square of filter paper. Put one tablet in the centre of the moist area. Flow two drops of water on to the tablet.

Negative Reaction. When no blue colour appears within two minutes.

Positive Reaction. When blood is present it will be recognised by the diffuse blue colour developing around the tablet within two minutes. The stronger the colour and the quicker the change, the greater is the amount of blood present.

2. Hemastix. Test for blood in the urine

REQUIREMENTS. Reagent strip. Colour chart.

METHOD. The urine must be clean and free from contaminants Mix the urine well before testing, to disperse any sediment. Dip the test end into the urine and remove immediately. Compare with colour chart exactly 30 seconds later. A blue colour on the test end will indicate the presence of blood.

3. Guaiac Test

REQUIREMENTS. Tincture of Guaiacum. Ozonic ether. Test tube. Pipette with rubber bulb.

METHOD. Place one inch urine in the test tube and add one to two drops of fresh tincture of Guaiacum. Add one-half inch of ozonic ether by dropping it slowly down the side of the test tube. A blue ring develops if blood is present.

A more reliable test is microscopic examination of a centrifuged specimen of urine.

TESTS FOR BILIRUBIN

Purpose : Detection of liver disease, haemolytic disease. etc.

1. Ictotest

REQUIREMENTS. Ictotest reagent tablets. Pipette with rubber bulb. Special test mat.

METHOD. Place five drops of urine on a square of the special test mat. Put one tablet on the centre of the moistened area. Place two drops of water on to the tablet with the pipette.

A negative reaction shows no bluish colour change within thirty seconds. Any change of colour to pink or red should be ignored.

A positive reaction is demonstrated when the mat around the tablet turns bluish-purple within thirty seconds. The amount of bilirubin present is proportional to the speed and intensity of the colour change.

2. Iodine Test

REQUIREMENTS. Tincture of iodine. Test tube. Pipette with rubber bulb.

METHOD. Tincture of iodine is diluted with an equal amount of water. This solution is then poured slowly down the side of the test tube containing 5 ml. of urine. A green ring will form if bilirubin is present.

TEST FOR PUS

Purpose : Detection of infection in the renal tract.

The presence of pus in the urine is best detected by microscopic examination; chemical tests are most unreliable.
A large quantity of pus in the urine can be detected using liquor potassae.

REQUIREMENTS. Liquor potassae. Two test tubes.

METHOD. Pour 2 in. of urine into a test tube and add 1 in. liquor potassae. Slowly pour urine from one tube to another. In the presence of sufficient pus the mixture will become ropy.

TEST FOR PHENYLKETONURIA

Purpose : Detection of phenylketonuria.

REQUIREMENTS. Phenistix with colour scale.

METHOD. Dip the end of the Phenistix in urine and remove immediately. Alternatively, press the end against the wet napkin. Compare the colour of dipped end with the colour scale after thirty seconds.
Negative. No grey or grey-green colour on the stick.
Positive. A colour change on the stick ranging from grey to deep grey-green occurs within thirty seconds.

The test is considered unreliable if carried out before the infant is six weeks old. A false positive result yielding a less stable green colour can be due to p-hydroxyphenylpyruvic acid in the urine. This occurs in tyrocinosis.

FERRIC CHLORIDE TEST

Purpose : Detection of phenylketonuria.

REQUIREMENTS. Ferric chloride 5 or 10 per cent aqueous solution.

METHOD. The urine must be acidified. 5 ml. of acidified urine is placed into a test tube and a few drops of the 5 or 10 per cent aqueous solution of ferric chloride is added. In the presence of phenylpyruvic acid a green colour will develop within 2-3 minutes.

BIBLIOGRAPHY

Ames Company: *Routine Urine Tests.*
Blenkison, C. H. (1967). Peritoneal dialysis. *Nurs. Times*, **68**, 578.
Garb, S. & Sporne, P. (1961). *Nurse's Manual of Laboratory Tests.*
  London: Heinemann.
Hutchison, J. H. (1967). *Practical Paediatric Problems*, 2nd ed. London:
  Lloyd-Luke.
Knowles, E. J. (1967). Peritoneal dialysis at six months. *Nurs. Times*,
  67, 1655.
Roper, N. (1966). *Livingstone's Dictionary for Nurses*, 12th ed. Edin-
  burgh: Livingstone.
Thomson, W. A. R. (1966). *Calling the Laboratory*, 2nd ed. Edinburgh:
  Livingstone.

CHAPTER XVIII

ORTHOPAEDIC NURSING OF CHILDREN

Care of children in splints; Jones pressure bandage; application of skin extension; application of splints; straight and abduction frame; plaster of Paris; Barlow's and Craig's divaricators.

ORTHOPAEDIC conditions which are found in a children's ward involve the bones, joints, muscles and soft tissues of the growing child. They include such deformities as lordosis, scoliosis and kyphosis, injury to bone through trauma or infection, and congenital deformities.

Long term immobilisation may be a necessary part of treatment and unless these children are given adequate means to get rid of their excess energy, both mental and physical, certain problems arise. They become very easily frustrated, have temper tantrums and rages or become moody and withdrawn. It is in an effort to prevent such occurrences that it can be truly said that the orthopaedic ward in a hospital is quite the noisiest one but usually the happiest one. It calls for ingenuity in planning to keep these children occupied. The physiotherapist, occupational therapist, and school teacher, together with the nursing and medical staff have a vital part to play. The problem of the child receiving long term care in an acute surgical ward where he can see children coming and going with monotonous regularity is even greater, and much careful planning on the part of the staff is required to ensure that his days are fully occupied and that he is kept happy and contented. The importance of regular, frequent visits by the parents cannot be overemphasised, and when this is not possible, a substitute visitor should be found.

The parents of such a child who is going to be cared for at home require help and guidance in understanding the child's special problems, and in this situation the health visitor and the family doctor can be of great assistance. No child will be happy who is not allowed some measure of independence. Methods must be found to enable him whenever possible to feed himself, read his own books, and to make and create. Singing is a wonderful way of relieving feelings and should be encouraged. Equipment should be adapted to suit individual needs and requires constant reviewing. Much research is carried out and new ways are found to help the handicapped children and make them more independent. Their courage and perseverance need all the help and encouragement that can be given to them.

Care of Children in Splints

1. OCCUPATION. This has been dealt with in the introductory note.

2. OBSERVATION. Constant vigilance is essential so that corrective appliances are maintained in the position in which they have been placed. Pressure and friction causing redness and pain or poor alignment must be reported, treated, or corrected. This is not only important for the child confined to bed but also while he is up and about. Detection of abnormalities will be simplified if the nurse is already familiar with the normal appearance, poise, balance and alignment of the healthy child at rest, at play and in action. It is very important, particularly in the initial phase, when the active child is confined to bed, to observe the amount of urine passed and the regularity of bowel movements. The fluid intake should be adequate and the diet contain fruit and roughage to ensure regular bowel actions. Vomiting too can be very troublesome and should it occur it must be reported. In an effort to prevent vomiting, meals may be given in small quantities but more frequently.

3. FEEDING. Hot plates must not be placed on paralysed limbs. Sensation may be totally absent and a severe burn may result. By raising the head with a small pillow, the position of the child may be altered during feeding to permit independent manipulation of a cup or plate. Special cups or feeders may be necessary to make drinking easier. Adequate fluid intake should be maintained, in order to prevent the formation of stones in the renal pelvis. This can occur where children have to be kept lying in bed for a long period, which prevents kidneys from excreting liberated calcium salts.

4. SANITARY ROUNDS. Two nurses are required to insert and remove bedpans from a child who is being treated by traction. The external genital area must be cleaned after each sanitary round. Where the foot of the bed is elevated, urine may trickle upwards. To prevent this happening, the child should be assisted to take

up the best possible position to urinate. This can be achieved by supporting the pelvis and holding the urinal (see nursing care for patient with a Thomas's bed splint).

5. CARE OF APPLIANCES. Appliances, walking machines, and wheel chairs are inspected daily for wear and tear and if necessary should be sent for repair immediately. Crutches are examined to make sure that they are safe for use and of the correct size, as children quickly outgrow these. Padded back splints require regular examination so that sores are not caused by exposed edges. Any appliance worn by a child with a paralysed limb requires the utmost care and attention because the child is unlikely to complain. Leather which becomes continuously contaminated with urine or faeces will harden and crack readily causing excoriation of the skin. Such leather should be treated frequently with leather soap and thoroughly dried. If necessary it may be covered with some waterproofing material. Spirit or other lotions which harden leather should not be used.

6. CHILDREN WHO ARE ALLOWED UP. Here the nurses' duties are to make sure that (a) the child walks and sits correctly with the appliance, (b) that the appliance is in the correct position, and (c) in all cases constant encouragement is necessary and help must always be available to allay fears. Toys such as tricycles are of tremendous help as exercising machines.

Advice to Parents

When the child is ready to go home, the following points should be discussed with the parents regarding the type of appliance the child is to have.

To avoid tripping and to make manipulation of the appliance safe, obstacles such as rugs should not be on the floor.

To encourage walking and crawling activities, space should be made available. This may not be easy where housing conditions are poor, and some arrangement will have to be made so that the exercise can be carried out.

Advice can be given regarding the type of toy which will be of benefit to the child and also amuse him; e.g., tricycle.

When the child is allowed home with a plaster of Paris splint, the following points should be made clear :

The plaster must be kept dry.

The plaster must be kept free from cracks. If cracks are present, the hospital should be notified. Meanwhile the child should be kept in bed until the plaster has been repaired. This applies particularly to hip and leg plasters.

If the child has been treated as an emergency, as in cases of fracture, and allowed home, the parents must be told what to watch for and when to notify the hospital authorities immediately.

1. Circulation—the limb must be pink and warm to the touch.

2. Swelling—this may persist for 24 hours but should not increase.

3. Pain—should gradually become less.

4. Loss of movement—the child should be able to move fingers and toes.

5. Irritation.

Children must be prevented from placing foreign bodies; e.g., buttons and pennies, into the plaster, which could easily cause pressure sores. If the plaster has been applied to a leg the child must not be allowed to bear weight on it for 72 hours.

LIFTING A CHILD IN HIP SPICA. After the first 48 hours, once a hip spica is dry, it is important that the child should spend at least four hours of the day lying on his abdomen. This adds variety to his position and the movement helps to prevent the formation of renal calculi. Turning the child requires great care. Support is necessary under the hip and the upper part of the leg. If the lower part of the plaster is lifted it may cause cracking of the plaster below the knee.

EXERCISE. Muscles will soon lose their tone if not exercised and the mother should be shown what exercises are necessary. Wriggling the toes of the affected limb and vigorous exercises of the unaffected limb, will help greatly when the time comes to walk again.

TOILET ARRANGEMENTS. The mother should be shown how bedpans and urinals are placed in the correct position and the child should not be sent home until suitable receptacles are available.

APPLICATION OF A JONES PRESSURE BANDAGE

This bandage is used in traumatic conditions affecting the knee, and is applied after a cartilage operation or any operation on the knee. It gives support to the knee and by its pressure has control of swelling. The flexible nature of the material used in bandaging the joint allows slight movement, roughly 5-10°.

REQUIREMENTS. Cotton wool—one roll. Crepe bandage 6 in. wide. Adhesive tape 1 in. wide.

METHOD. A thick layer of wool is wound around the knee. Three firm turns are made directly over the joint with the crepe bandage. This should cover 3-6 in. below and above the joint. Another layer of cotton wool is then applied and three more turns are made around the joint. This is repeated until the bandage is finished. Before returning the child to bed the circulation must be satisfactory. Safety pins should not be applied to the bandage as children are apt to play with them. Adhesive tape of suitable length should be used, but it must not encircle the limb.

APPLICATION OF SKIN EXTENSION

The application of skin extension may be required for fixed traction or for use with weights and pulley, in the treatment of the following:

1. Perthes disease of the hip—traction frees the head of the femur from the acetabulum.

2. Frame fixation for aiding reduction of the congenital dislocation of the hip.

3. To reduce a fracture of the femur in conjunction with the Thomas splint.

4. To gently reduce contracture of the knee by applying the traction below the knee.

5. To rest a diseased hip or limb.

6. It is applied to a baby's legs when the gallows extension is used to reduce a fracture of the femur.

Action of Long Axis Traction

When the adhesive extension is applied to the skin and fixed or anchored by the tapes to the end of the bed splint, or when the tapes with weights added pass over a pulley, the pull is transferred from the skin to the muscles and then to the bone. Therefore if applied to the legs in preparation for reducing the congenital dislocation of the hip, the head of the femur is gently pulled downwards nearer the acetabulum. If applied to the legs in the treatment of Perthes disease of the hip, it frees the head of the femur from bearing weight, enabling it to rest.

REQUIREMENTS:

THE BED. The bed is prepared with a fracture board beneath the mattress. A cradle is necessary to protect the feet. An elevator is placed under the bed end to provide countertraction. Countertraction is the pull of the patient's body weight away from the elevated bed end. Pulleys are attached to the end of the bed for sliding traction. A hook may be used in place of the pulley if fixed traction is ordered.

SHAVING TRAY (if necessary):

1. Water repellent sheet.
2. Container with cotton wool.
3. Container with warm water.
4. Soap in a soap dish.
5. Container with razor and blades.
6. Scissors.
7. Receptacle for disposable items.
8. Receptacle for salvage.

METHOD. Gentle handling of the limb is essential and a second nurse may be required to aid the necessary movements. The water repellent sheet is placed beneath the limb. Soap is applied liberally all over the limb. The skin is then held taut and the hair removed by drawing the razor downwards in the direction of the hair growth. There should be no cuts or scratches. The limb is then washed and dried thoroughly.

TRAY OR TROLLEY TO CONTAIN THE FOLLOWING REQUIREMENTS:

1. Tape measure.
2. Elastoplast extension plaster 2 in. or 3 in. wide.
3. Scissors.
4. Anklets made of lint $\frac{3}{4}$ in. in depth.
5. Crepe bandages 4 in. and 6 in. wide.
6. Wooden spreader.
7. Green cord, lengths of 2 yards each.
8. Lampwick $\frac{1}{4}$ in. wide and 18 in. in length (4 lengths required).
9. Needle and strong thread.
10. Bowl with cotton wool.
11. Toggles.

MEASUREMENTS REQUIRED:

1. Measure the distance between the great trochanter and the lateral malleolus and subtract ¾ in. or less according to the age of the child.
2. Measure the inside of the leg but subtract 2 in. or 3 in. so that the extension plaster does not adhere to the external genital area.
3. Measure round the limb ¾ in. above the malleolus.

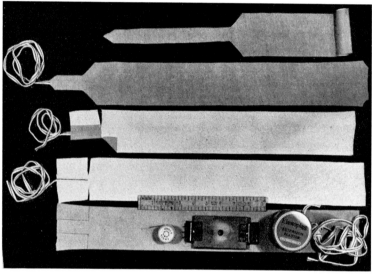

FIG. 73
Preparation of adhesive extension for fixed and sliding traction

To Make Extension for Fixed Traction

The extension plaster is rolled out on a scrupulously clean surface. The required lengths are measured, allowing 1½ in. more adhesive plaster to enclose the lampwick. The adhesive plaster is cut into, to a depth of 1 in. on both sides, 1½ in. from the end. This leaves 1 in. in the centre. The end of the lampwick is placed in the centre and the cut sides are folded over it. This is then stitched securely. The ends of the approximated plaster are then fixed neatly back. The prepared extension should be held up by the lampwick ends and neatly notched on both sides to ensure better fixation. The lengths for the inner and outer parts of the limb should be clearly marked. They are then hung on the end of a table or trolley free from other materials to which they might adhere (Fig. 73),

A skin traction kit is available which simplifies both preparation and application of skin traction. It consists of the following:

1. Elastoplast extension plaster.
2. Elastocrepe bandage.
3. A spreader which is firmly bonded to the plaster.
4. Soft foam lining to cushion the ankle joint and sides of the foot against pressure.
5. Traction cords.

The adhesive surfaces of the kit are covered with a plastic protective backing, avoiding handling long lengths of sticky plaster. It can be used for treatment on the Thomas splint, weight traction and skin traction.

To Make Extension for Weight and Pulley Traction

The method is the same, but instead of allowing $1\frac{1}{2}$ in. in excess of the required length for the limb, 8 in. is allowed. No lampwick is necessary as the 3 ply 8 in. length acts as a strap to secure extensions to the spreader. It is cut in the same way as previously mentioned.

If used for a baby the extension should be cut to shape along the contours above the ankle.

To Apply Long Axis Traction

If the child is old enough, an explanation of the appliance should be given. The anklet is applied with an additional $\frac{1}{4}$ in. in width, but it should not be too tight. Fix with adhesive tape. The anklet should not have a selvedge, but a frayed edge which will allow for expansion or swelling of the limb if it has been injured.

A nurse then takes hold of the limb, cupping the heel in her hand, her fingers clasped just above the malleoli. A firm pull is maintained on the leg. This lessens the pain and if a fracture of the femur is being treated, it prevents movement of the fractured parts.

The inner extension is applied by adhering first $\frac{3}{4}$ in. above the malleolus and then smoothing the remainder all along the inside of the leg to within suitable distance of the external genital area.

There must be no creases or folds. The outer extension is applied in the same manner. If the extensions overlap at the back of the leg, care must be taken to remove creases to obtain perfect smoothness.

Before applying the bandage the following should be noted :
  1. The patella should be free and uncovered.
  2. The crest of the tibia should be visible.
  3. The malleoli should be protected.

The patella is then protected with a flick of cotton wool and commencing at the ankle, the crepe bandage is applied evenly. A bandage is applied in a figure of eight to below the knee and is then continued with spiral turns over the thigh. It is fixed with adhesive tape of 2 in. length. The circulation must not be impeded by the firm bandaging or by the bandage covering the dorsum of the foot.

Method Used in Weight and Pulley Traction

The buckles of the wooden spreader are fixed between the ends of the adhesive extensions. Sufficient room is left to allow the foot to move and exercise. There must be no pressure from the spreader and toggles near the sole of the foot. The extension cord is folded in the centre and pushed as a loop through the hole in the spreader. The loop of extension cord is then secured with a spatula and adhesive. The cord is then placed over the pulley at the foot of the bed and the correct weight added. It is important to make certain that the weights are secure.

In both cases a cradle is placed over the child's feet to take the weight of the bedclothes, thus freeing the feet for exercises and freedom of movement. An elevator is placed under the foot of the bed to raise it and aid countertraction.

CARE OF THE CHILD. While lying on his back the child is taught how to play, keeping his shoulder on the bed in order to maintain traction and assist in maintaining the correct position. The nurse passing up and down the ward must observe that the appliance is fulfilling its function; i.e., the weights must not lie on the floor or be obstructed in any way either by knots in the cord or by being caught in the pulley.

In conditions other than fractures the crepe bandage is removed daily to allow inspection of the limb. Hyperextension of the knee and chafing of the malleoli must be prevented. The foot should be of good colour, move freely, and the heel must not press into the mattress.

Gallows Traction

This form of traction is employed in the treatment of fracture of the femur in children up to $1\frac{1}{2}$ years of age. (Fig. 74)

The same materials are required as in skin traction with the addition of a metal frame. Weights are usually not required but should be prepared in case the doctor wishes to apply weight and pulley traction.

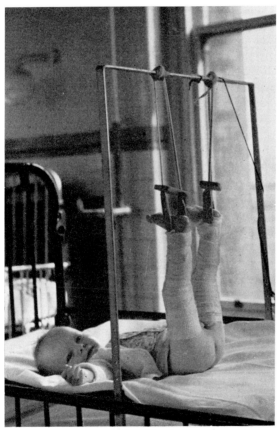

FIG. 74
Gallows traction

METHOD:

1. See application of skin extension.
2. The legs are raised and fixed with the lampwick to the horizontal bar of the frame. The buttocks should be just clear of the bed and the hips flexed to a right angle. A folded napkin is placed between the thighs and a small blanket can be pinned around the two legs.

Nursing care presents few problems and the small child is usually very comfortable while lying in this position. Pressure areas are easily treated and napkin changes readily carried out. Special care is necessary when changing the napkin and treating the buttocks. The nurse should place her hands under the child's axillae and pull him gently upwards and backwards. This will maintain the position of traction. Areas such as the scapulae and the back of the head require attention to prevent chafing due to friction. The hair should be brushed and combed regularly to prevent matting. When bottle feeding the small infant, the head and shoulders should be raised during feeding and the infant helped to expel any air he may have swallowed. The toddler can have a pillow under his head during meal times and a spouted feeder or beaker for drinking.

The toddler must be given adequate toys to play with; these should be placed within easy reach of the child and every opportunity used to play and talk with him.

The child may be discharged home on a gallows stretcher frame. Clear instructions must be given to the parents regarding the care of the child, maintenance of traction and correct position. Both parents should be shown how to handle the child and be encouraged to nurse him under guidance, while still in hospital.

Head Traction

Where there is inter-locking of the inter-articular facets of the vertebrae, this form of traction is applied. It can occur to patients with a dislocation of the cervical spine.

REQUIREMENTS:

1. Bed with fracture board.
2. Elevator—to raise the head of the bed.
3. Bedcage.

4. Pulley.
5. Weights (up to 10 lb.).
6. Leather head band with chin straps.
7. Metal bar with hooks for attachment of a head band and traction cord.

METHOD. The pulley is fitted behind the top of the bed in line with the patient's head. A pillow should not be used as it interrupts the traction. The child lies in the supine position.

The chin is cupped in the leather part made for it in the head piece and the side chin straps are buckled into the head band strap which passes under the base of the skull. The side pieces press up the side of the face allowing no pressure on the ears, and are hooked on to the metal bar which supports the cord passing over the pulley holding the weights.

NURSING CARE. The chin requires great care. Only good quality soap should be used. The chin is washed with soap and water and dried thoroughly three times a day. At other times it is sufficient to undo the chin strap for a few minutes.

During meal times, a napkin should be tucked temporarily under the chin covering the leather. A leather chin strap which has been allowed to get damp or soiled will cause friction and lead to a break in the continuity of the skin accompanied by severe pain. Treatment may then have to be discontinued.

The heels and buttocks require regular care. The child should have a good view from his bed and this can be facilitated by the suitable positioning of a mirror. Toys and books should be readily available to keep the child occupied and amused. Movement of the legs is encouraged and balloon and ball games provide much happiness while lying in this position.

APPLICATION OF SPLINTS

Arm Splint for the Correction of Erb's Paralysis

Erb's paralysis is caused at birth. It is due to traction injury to the fifth and sixth cervical nerve roots. There is paralysis of the deltoid, biceps, supraspinatus, intraspinatus and the supinators of the forearm. The arm hangs by the side of his body and is flaccid, showing the characteristic 'porter's hand'.

If the injury has been slight, there may be some bleeding into the nerve sheath, and spontaneous recovery occurs.

All injuries require rest. A temporary measure is to pin the cuff of the sleeve of the baby's gown to the pillow by taking the arm upwards over the baby's head and fixing comfortably until splintage is applied. Various types of splints may be used. Kramer wire is simple and effective or an acrylic splint may be made. The aim of splintage is to hold the limb in full external rotation and abduction at the shoulder, right-angled flexion of the elbow and full supination of the forearm.

PREPARATION FOR SPLINTAGE USING KRAMER WIRE.

REQUIREMENTS:

1. Kramer wire.
2. Wire cutters.
3. Scissors.
4. Orthopaedic adhesive felt.
5. 2 in. crepe bandage.
6. Cotton wool for axillae.
7. Talcum powder.
8. Adhesive tape.

PREPARATION AND APPLICATION OF THE SPLINT. The positioning and initial application of the splint is carried out by the doctor. The arm is abducted just short of full abduction at right angles to the trunk. The elbow is flexed in a semi- or mid-position. The forearm is fully supinated and the wrist is dorsiflexed. A cotton wool pad is then placed in the axilla and the padded splint is applied.

DAILY NURSING CARE. The axilla is examined for chafing. The arm is washed with soap and water, dried thoroughly and dusted with talcum powder. The splint is then reapplied.

Physiotherapy is given daily. This is commenced at once to prevent contractures. Each joint is put through a full range of its own movements.

AFTER CARE GIVEN TO THE BABY BY THE MOTHER. The mother is instructed how to change and re-apply the splint and to encourage abduction and external rotation as the child grows. A coloured ball or rattle which the baby can see will act as inducement to move the arm affected and encourage co-operation. The sound arm may be slipped out of the sleeve and lightly bandaged to the body for

short periods, this will allow movement and exercise of the paralysed arm.

The Thomas's Bed Splint

This splint provides immobilisation and traction and maintains
extension. It may be used for either leg. The ring is shaped to
fit the upper part of the limb, the higher side of the ring fits the
outer aspect of the thigh.

It is used for the following purposes :

(a) To immobilise and maintain extension in the fracture of a
femur, and sometimes in the fracture of tibia and fibula.
(b) To rest an infected knee where, if necessary, the knee can
be clearly exposed for examination without disturbing the
limb.
(c) It provides immobilisation for diseased or infected parts, or
inflammatory lesions of the lower limb.

REQUIREMENTS FOR FIXED TRACTION OR WEIGHT AND PULLEY
TRACTION:

1. Bed or cot.
2. Fracture board beneath the mattress.
3. Elevator.
4. Cradle.
5. Hook, to fix in abduction on the cot, placed 6 in. above the
mattress, or pulley fixed in position of abduction to the right
or left according to which limb is being treated.

REQUIREMENTS FOR THE TROLLEY (Fig. 75). The trolley is laid
with requirements as for long axis skin traction plus:

1. One block of wood 8 in. high.
2. Foot cradle.
3. Calico bandages 6 in. wide to be used as slings on the splint.
4. Three safety pins (curved).
5. Cotton wool for padding beneath the head of the tibia.
6. Two pieces of cotton wool the length of the limb.
7. Inch tape.
8. Orthoband or wool bandage.

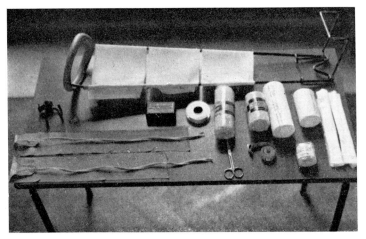

Fig. 75
Preparation for fixed long axis traction and Thomas's bed splint

Before the splint is applied, the patient's limb is measured in the following way:

1. Round the thigh at the level of the abductor tendon (groin).
2. From the lower end of the upper fractured bone to the heel and 6 in. or 8 in. are added to allow for tying traction tapes and application of foot cradle. Note whether the splint is required for the right or left limb.

The splint, which must be of the correct width and size, is then checked with the measurements and first tried on the sound leg. Extra width should be allowed, as swelling may occur. The three slings, which are made from calico bandage, are placed on the splint and fastened with curved safety pins. These pins are placed on the outer side of the limb for easy adjustment and fastened under the calico slings. The prepared splint is finally covered with Orthoband to prevent pressure on the leg.

APPLICATION OF THE SPLINT. Sedation may be required if the limb is painful. This should be given at a stated time prior to the application. The patient is taken to the dressing room in his bed and, if he is old enough, a simple explanation should be given. Any temporary or first aid appliance is removed gently while the limb is held with gentle but firm traction. If necessary, the limb is cleaned with soap and water and dried thoroughly.

Long axis skin traction is applied first (see application of skin extension).

1. If a weight and pulley traction is to be used, the extension plaster with an additional 6 in. or 8 in. length is required.
2. If fixed traction is to be used the extension plaster with the lampwick fixed to it is required, plus an additional 1½ in. of extension plaster.

Some surgeons use the beginning of 4 in. bandage to protect the malleolus and to correct a tendency to deformity and, in this case, the anklet is not necessary. The crepe bandage is commenced in a figure of eight at the ankle as far as the knee, then continued spiral fashion over the thigh. The splint is then handed to the doctor or his assistant with the slings pinned to the outside and covered with a length of cotton wool. It is gently guided over the foot and the ring is carried up the leg and fitted comfortably around the thigh. If a fracture is being treated, a doctor holds and maintains a pull on the limb after he has manually reduced the fracture.

A pad of cotton wool is then placed just above the popliteal space to allow 5° flexion, and near the fracture site according to the need for correction of displacement. The lampwick is tied securely and the end of the splint now rests temporarily on a block of wood. A 6 in. bandage is applied over the splint and care should be taken to commence the bandage in a position that in no way interferes with the exercises of the foot.

The limb should be resting on the sling, and two-thirds of the limb exposed above the Thomas's splint. The appearance of the limb should show the normal bowing of the thigh. A foot piece is applied and fixed with adhesive. A cover is placed over the child exposing the splinted leg. To keep the exposed foot warm, a woollen sock is applied. The Thomas's splint is now fixed on the hook which has been placed 6 in. above the matttess.

NURSING CARE: SANITARY ROUND. A nurse should take a warmed bedpan to the bedside and a second nurse should assist her. They should then fold back the bedclothes, the assisting nurse places her hands round the child's pelvis, her thumbs resting on the anterior superior iliac spine, and her fingers over the lumbar region. She should ask the child to draw up his sound knee to right angles and press his foot into the bed. She then gently raises the pelvis upwards, maintaining gentle traction towards the head of the bed. The first nurse now places the bedpan in position and remains with the child until urine or faeces has been passed. Later, the child can be trained to use both utensils at the same time (Fig. 76).

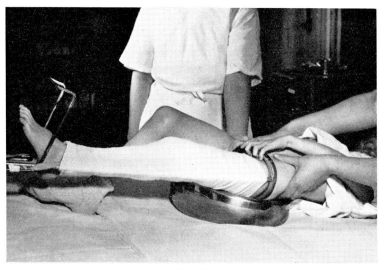

FIG. 76
Placing a child with a Thomas's splint on a bedpan

DAILY INSPECTION OF THE LIMB. The child should be asked to exercise his foot each time the routine toilet round takes place and at bedmaking time.

Daily inspection is imperative.

The whole length of the limb in the bed splint is examined for the following:

1. The ring must remain in the correct position, leather must be dry and the skin free from sores and redness. There must be no pressure on the iliac spine.
2. Absence of pain behind and above the heel.
3. The malleoli must be free from friction.
4. The movement of the foot should be normal and painless. There must be no sign of drop foot.
5. Traction must be maintained and must never be released unless by a doctor.

Thereafter the bedclothes are replaced, and care must be taken to ensure that they do not cause pressure on the foot.

PHYSIOTHERAPY. During immobilisation in a Thomas's bed splint (or fixation in plaster of paris) it is vitally important to maintain muscle tone, especially of the larger muscles which will tend to waste very quickly; e.g., the quadriceps. In conditions affecting the knee joint, the child is taught to do a static contraction of the quadriceps muscles within the Thomas's bed splint (or within the plaster of paris), i.e. the muscles contract and relax without the joint moving. This is sufficient to maintain muscle tone and assist the circulation of blood in the limb.

After removal of a bed splint, the physiotherapist will give formal exercises and will state when the child is ready to walk. The physiotherapist is with the child for short periods only, so it is important for the nurse to encourage him to exercise his limbs. He should be bathed in a large bath, preferably in the morning, where he can splash and exercise his limbs under water and greatly enjoy the progress he is making. Assistance from another nurse may be required to lift him carefully out of the bath. Help must be available until movements are less painful and he is more confident. When necessary the nurse should provide a walking chair, and a wheel chair given for short periods will add greatly to his delight.

COMPLICATION WHICH MAY OCCUR.

DROP FOOT. When a foot cannot voluntarily be raised to the normal angle, it is said to be a drop foot.

It may be due to:

1. The Thomas's bed splint causing pressure over the external popliteal nerve.
2. Bandages applied too firmly, leading to injury to the external popliteal nerve.
3. The weight of the bedclothes.
4. Failure to encourage and supervise exercises.

Denis Browne's Foot Splints for Talipes

Denis Browne's foot splints are used for correction of talipes equino varus. This deformity is present at birth. Three distinct components of the deformity may be recognised:

1. Plantar flexion of the foot at the ankle so that the foot points downwards.
2. Inversion of the foot so that the soles of the feet face each other.
3. Abduction of the foot.

Treatment is commenced as soon as possible after birth, preferably within eight days. After the feet have been photographed, they are manipulated daily. As soon as a partial correction has been obtained, a single Denis Browne splint can be fitted and when a little further improvement has taken place, a pair of Denis Browne splints with bar are applied.

REQUIREMENTS:

1. Prepared Denis Browne splints.
2. Transverse bar.
3. Screws and bolts.
4. Spanner, correct size to fit screws and bar to the foot piece.
5. Elastoplast 1 in. wide and 3 yds. long.
6. $\frac{1}{4}$ inch squares of adhesive felt $\frac{1}{4}$ inch thick.
7. Table covered with a sheet and a pillow.

TRAY WITH THE FOLLOWING:

1. Cotton wool.
2. 3 containers for methylated ether, methylated spirit and Cetavlon.
3. Soap in a soap dish.
4. Large bowl with warm water.
5. Towel.
6. Receptacle for soiled cotton wool.

POSITION OF THE BABY FOR MANIPULATION. The baby is placed comfortably at the foot of the table with a small pillow placed below his head. The nurse separates the legs and grasps the calf of the leg in both hands, thereby protecting the knee from strain. The inversion and abduction of the foot is corrected first and the plantar-flexion last.

APPLICATION OF THE SPLINT. The surgeon places a small piece of adhesive felt over the talus. The sole piece is then applied to the foot and with 1 in. Elastoplast it is bandaged into the position correcting the forefoot adduction. The leg pieces project outwards from the leg. These, when bandaged to the leg, pull the foot into eversion. The sole pieces are then fitted to the cross bar pointing outwards in as much external rotation as possible.

The toes should be pink and, after removal of digital pressure, the skin should flush quickly with blood. If the toes are not pink the feet should be elevated, and should this fail, the bar between the splints can be removed. As a final resort it may be necessary to remove the splints. The baby is free to kick and be active. The splints are kept in the corrected position day and night.

Once over-correction has been obtained usually after 10-14 days the child is allowed home, often in a plaster for one month, though this is not essential. Thereafter, the baby attends every two weeks for remanipulation of the feet and re-application of Denis Browne splints.

ADVICE TO THE MOTHER. The mother is asked to observe the toes and contact the hospital at once should anything abnormal occur. It should be explained to her that there may be some swelling of the toes, but they should be pink and flush readily after removal of digital pressure. Gross swelling and discolouration must be reported at once.

When the child shows determination to stand on his feet, about 10-12 months old, Denis Browne splints are discontinued and he is put into boots, with heels reduced and a raise on the outer part of the sole—this puts the child in a calcaneo valgus position each time he stands on his feet. The parents are taught to manipulate the feet into that position daily and put the child into boots with correcting bar at night.

THE STRAIGHT FRAME

The straight frame provides rest for children suffering from tuberculosis of the spine or other diseases requiring enforced immobilisation. It supplies a means of aiding correction of deformity of the spine, hip or legs, by positioning the body while undergoing prolonged treatment.

This frame has two longitudinal metal bars which extend from the nipple line to the gluteal fold. The lowest inch of the bars is curved backward to receive the ischial tuberosity. Extending from this point two other longitudinal bars are joined at an angle of 15°; these support the legs to just above the ankles. The lower bars are joined by a cross bar and are united to the knock-knee bars by crutches in which the ankles rest. The nipple and pelvic bars are made of malleable metal which can be moulded to fit the patient's body. These are riveted to the main part. Knock-knee bars which are made from malleable metal can be bent to lie in the long axis of the legs. A head piece is screwed to the longitudinal bars. This is a metal framework fashioned to fit the back of the head comfortably. A straight head piece has a flat surface and a sunken head piece a hollowed surface.

The saddle is made of the best quality leather and placed over the metal framework. The appropriate parts should correspond with the identical parts on the metal frame. The tension of the stuffing within the saddle is important to the patient's comfort. It is evenly packed with lambswool. The saddle supports the trunk from the seventh cervical vertebra to the tip of the coccyx. The leg pieces support the parts from the tip of the coccyx and the legs to below the knee joint. The saddle is fixed to the metal frame by tapes which are threaded through the back of the saddle.

The child is kept secure by means of strong leather belts which are attached to the back of the saddle.

The nursing care regarding feeding and sanitary round, is the same as for a child lying in a plaster cast. A plaster of Paris turning case is made for the child so that he can be removed from the frame to enable inspection and treatment of pressure areas. It also permits cleaning of the saddle. This may be done by removing all dried particles of excreta or foreign material with a wooden spatula or other blunt instrument. The leather is then washed with leather soap and dried thoroughly before it is polished with a soft, clean cloth. The metal parts are cleaned with soap and water. Exposed metal parts which may be in contact with the child are covered with adhesive felt. Groin straps should be plentiful and any soiled ones replaced immediately. At the same time, the nurse must check that all tapes and belts are securely attached and able to fulfil their purpose.

Preparation and Method for Turning a Child Nursed on a Straight Frame

REQUIREMENTS:

1. Plaster of Paris turning case.

2. Belts with buckles.
3. Bathing blankets.
4. ½in. wide tape, needles and strong white thread to repair or strengthen the tapes.
5. Soap in a soap dish.
6. Nail brush.
7. Bath towel.
8. Brush and comb.
9. Leather soap.
10. Wooden spatulae.
11. Bowl with cotton wool.
12. Bowl with gauze swabs.
13. Receptacle for used cotton wool and swabs.

METHOD. A simple explanation should be given to the child of what is about to happen and the bed prepared as for a blanket bath. Three nurses are required to turn the child.

The child is lifted on his frame to the side of the bed and the nipple and pelvis bars are undone. If weights are used, these are removed carefully. The bandages are removed and the child is undressed. The turning case is fitted over his trunk and legs while he is still in the frame. The belts are fitted over the lumbar region, trunk, one under each axilla and around each leg. The belts are buckled firmly to the sides to ensure the child's safety while in mid-air.

The nurses now stand at each side of the bed and lift the child clear of the bed. He is turned in mid-air and comes down to rest in his shell face downwards. The straps are unbuckled and the frame removed without delay. It is important to ascertain that the child is free from dizziness before commencing with any treatment. The child's back is then inspected and the condition of the skin observed. The spine is examined for any changes such as an increase in a kyphosis. The whole area including the back of the legs and heels, is then treated with soap and water and thoroughly dried. While the child is in this position, it is a good opportunity to wash his hair.

When the procedure is completed, the saddle and frame are fixed into position again. The method for turning is repeated by applying the frame over the body instead of the plaster of Paris shell.

THE ABDUCTION FRAME

This splint is used because it allows traction and counter-traction at the hip joint, and is useful in the treatment of congenital dislocation of the hip. It permits inspection of the parts and observation of alignment. It is made of the same materials as the straight frame and presents the same longitudinal bars, nipple bars, pelvic bars, knock-knee bars and crutches for the ankles. The cross bar is pierced with holes to adjust the leg pieces to the degree of abduction required. When adjusting the degree of abduction, the screws are removed and re-positioned in the required holes. The saddle is similar to that used with the straight

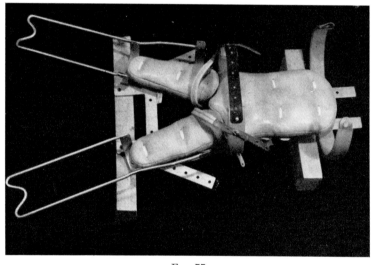

FIG. 77
Abduction frame

frame, except that the leg pieces are separated from the trunk but can be easily approximated and guided outwards when abduction is required (Fig. 77).

The incidence of congenital dislocation of the hip is eight times more frequent in girls than boys (Mason Brown, 1962). For this reason we use the feminine gender.

Abduction Frame Fixation

Frame fixation may be the treatment necessary to reduce congenital dislocation of hip. This allows for gradual reduction without the use of force. This method gives traction to and across the long axis of the limbs. It is effective if the head of the femur is not markedly displaced.

MEASUREMENTS FOR A FRAME. The same measurements are required for a straight and abduction frame:

1. From the nipple line to the gluteal fold.
2. From the gluteal fold to $1\frac{1}{2}$ in. above the malleoli.
3. Round the chest at the nipple line.
4. Round the pelvis.
5. From the gluteal fold to halfway between the trochanter and the crest of the ilium.

SADDLE:

6. From the 7th cervical vertebra to the coccyx.
7. From the coccyx to mid-calf.
8. Measure $\frac{1}{3}$ of the measurement of a fully expanded chest.
9. Take the mid-inguinal measurement, i.e. measure from the right femoral artery to the left femoral artery.

TO PREPARE A CHILD FOR FRAME FIXATION. The child should be shown the frame and given the saddle to feel. It should be explained to her that this is going to be her bed. The child is weighed before going on the frame. The bowels should be acting daily. The buttocks should be free from redness or abrasions.

The nurse should cover with adhesive felt the parts of the frame which are likely to come into contact with the child, and the metal parts which are not touching the body are covered with lengths of cotton strips. Sufficient space should be left between the legs for nursing purposes, otherwise the saddle will become soiled and hardened leather will cause sores on the buttocks which may become infected and lead to cessation of the treatment.

TO PLACE A CHILD ON A FRAME. A long axis skin traction is applied, using adhesive extension plaster with 18 in. length of lampwick attached. All clothes are removed and with assistance from two nurses, the child is placed on the frame. The coccyx should just overlap the point of the saddle and the pelvic bars should fit. The nipple bars should fit comfortably, and the groin straps should not be too tight. Three pillows are placed under the child's head to give greater comfort. The lampwick is then fixed to the frame at bow shaped end of the leg pieces. The nipple bars are then adjusted and tied. A light weight frock or jacket which fastens behind at the nape of the neck is put on the child. The chest is thus covered and the sides of the frock hang freely. No material should come between the skin and the saddle.

One nurse should stand at the side of the child and keep the pelvis evenly placed on the saddle of the frame. Another nurse places little cushions of cotton wool under the head of each tibia and a snippet of cotton wool over each patella before bandaging the limbs to the frame. The anterior superior iliac spine, the patella and the big toe should be in a straight line. Beginning at the lateral knock bar of the frame the limb is bandaged lightly to the leg pieces of the frame. Space is left in front of the ankles for movement and exercise of the feet. Extensions to the foot piece are then tightened.

GENERAL NURSING CARE OF THE CHILD. The child is nursed on a bed with a fracture board and an elevator raises the foot of the bed. If the child has not been trained to ask for a bedpan, a bedpan should be placed below her and a napkin placed over the vulva. Another napkin should be rolled and placed behind the bedpan. This will protect the wooden support of the frame from becoming saturated with urine should the child by chance or design displace the bedpan. The child should be given toys to play with and the nurse or other children should be encouraged to play games with the child. Talking and reading to the child are equally important and any tearful episode should be investigated and relieved.

The child is nursed for three days in this position and, on the fourth day, 3 lb. weight is added to the skin extension of each limb, this being maintained for the 5th and 6th day. On the 7th day abduction of the legs is commenced and 5° abduction is made every day until 90° abduction is obtained. Careful attention is paid to the adductors. If they are found to be tight, they are allowed to rest for a day or two; lanolin may be applied to the groin to loosen the skin. When 90° abduction is obtained, no further abduction is permitted. If a bilateral congenital dislocation of hip is being treated and the head of the femur stands away, cross pull may be applied and the groin straps removed. If the dislocation is unilateral, only one groin strap is removed from the affected side for the application of the pull.

DESCRIPTION OF A CROSS PULL. Cuffs made of leather are fitted round the upper thigh. A little metal ring is built into the cuff for the insertion of the cord, and is placed to the inside of the thigh. Eyelets are inserted on each side of the cuff. The cuff is secured by lacing, as one laces a corset. The cord passes from the ring in the cuff diagonally to the pulley opposite at the foot of the frame; on this end 3 lb. weights are applied. The pulley is fixed to the terminal end of the leg pieces of the frame.

The function of the cross pull in uncomplicated dislocations is to aid in bringing the head of the femur gradually nearer the acetabulum. Properly applied and maintained, this allows gentle and continuous traction. It is important to ensure that the weight of the bedclothes does not interfere with the cross pull traction. If this traction is not effective, it may be due to an abnormality such as a limbus. This can be revealed by an arthrogram.

DAILY NURSING CARE

1. The bandages should be removed and the limbs inspected.
2. The area over the malleoli must not be chafed or rubbed.
3. The feet must be of good colour and should move freely to perform their normal function.
4. The heels should not be allowed to press into the mattress.
5. Hyperextension of the knees must be prevented, this can be achieved by maintaining flexion of the knees at 5°.
6. Any swellings or deformities must be watched for and foot drop prevented by supporting the bedclothes by a bed cradle.

To TREAT THE BUTTOCKS. The pelvic belt is untied and the groin straps removed while the pelvic bars are gently pulled apart. A second nurse stands beside the child facing the feet, her hands around the pelvic girdle and her thumbs on the anterior superior iliac spines. The child is then lifted gently upwards allowing sufficient room for the nurse to insert a napkin under the buttocks covering and protecting the saddle.

The vulva and buttocks are washed with soap and water and care is taken to dry the skin thoroughly. Only a good quality soap should be used. On completion of toilet care, the pelvic bar is fitted across and the groin straps fixed into position.

P.N.P.—M

The nurse should train her eyes to glance over the child's body, especially the pelvis and the legs, to see that the cleft between the buttocks is centrally placed and just overhanging the frame, and that the coccyx is on the point of the saddle. The anterior superior spines must be level, and the anterior superior spine, patella and the big toe should be in a straight line or as near straight as can be allowed. It is sometimes necessary to coax the knee of the affected side gently into a position with the patella pointing to the ceiling.

To lift a patient, while on a frame with a head piece, from the bed to a table, the nurse stands beside the patient facing across the pelvis. With one hand on the cross bar, which joins the leg pieces of the frame, and the other on the securely fixed nipple bar, she lifts the frame and the patient to the required height.

If there is no head piece, she first arranges three pillows on the table and lifts the child on the frame by holding the cross bar with one hand, and cradling the top of the frame and the child's head with her other arm.

PLASTER OF PARIS

Plaster of Paris is a fine powder derived from calcium sulphate. When the dry powder is mixed with water, a chemical reaction takes place and the powder sets into a solid cake. Final hardening occurs by the drying off of excessive quantities of water. During setting it becomes warm. Prepared bandages must be kept absolutely dry and stored in damp-proof containers.

Plaster of Paris may be applied after the reduction of a fracture, or after the surgical treatment of a soft tissue wound, or to retain the position of a limb or spine following operation on a bone or joint.

PREPARATION OF THE CHILD. Limbs in older children are sometimes covered with cotton wool, stockinet or gauze, or the plaster may be applied directly to the skin. Bony prominences can be protected with orthopaedic felt, but in all cases a minimum of padding is usually used.

REQUIREMENTS:

1. Large rubber mackintosh sheets.
2. Two deep bowls or buckets containing water at 36·8°C or 98·4°F.
3. Plaster bandages, assorted sizes.

4. Orthopaedic felt.
5. 'Tubegauz' or stockinet.
6. Large plaster shears and small plaster cutters.
7. Strong scissors and plaster knife.
8. Tape measure.
9. Skin pencil.
10. Any special appliance such as a wooden rocking heel.

METHOD. The plaster bandage should be immersed in the water for approximately 10 seconds or until air bubbles cease to rise from it. It should never be squeezed while under the water as this expels much of the useful plaster. When the bandage is lifted out of the bowl, excessive water is removed by squeezing gently from the ends towards the middle. The plaster begins to set very quickly and if bandages are not used immediately, they become hard and caked. The 'cream' that remains at the bottom of the bowl can be used to fill the surface crevices of the cast and produce a smooth finish. A smooth plaster does not get dirty so quickly as a rough plaster. The palm of the hand should be used to support the limb and care taken to prevent the fingers pressing into the wet plaster causing a dent which could lead to a pressure sore.

To allow the plaster to dry, the child should be turned every two hours for small plaster casts, and every four hours for a hip spica. Artificial heat is not necessary and is not recommended because of the danger of the plaster cracking, but a free circulation of air is important. The whole limb must be supported if a hip spica and a full leg plaster have been applied, to prevent the plaster cracking at the groin. Weight-bearing should not be permitted for approximately 72 hours.

AFTER CARE.

1. CIRCULATION. The most important immediate complication to watch for is restriction of venous return. The fingers and toes must be left uncovered and inspected repeatedly during the first few hours. The following must be watched for and reported immediately:

(*a*) Swelling and loss of movement.
(*b*) Impairment or loss of touch sensation. This can be tested with a piece of cotton wool.
(*c*) Blueness.

(*d*) Pallor of nail-beds and failure to flush after applying digital pressure.

2. PREVENTION OF PRESSURE SORES. Pieces of cotton wool or other substances must not be stuffed in at the ends.

3. PAIN. This may be due to pressure ulcers developing where excessive pressure is applied to the skin.

4. IRRITATION. This may be due to skin reaction and can be very distressing.

5. CRACKS IN THE PLASTER. This will render the plaster useless and it is always advisable to renew the plaster rather than repair it.

Removal of Plaster Cast

This requires considerable physical effort and care must be taken not to injure the skin with plaster shears. Small bites must be taken and the blades kept clean. An explanation should be given to the child and reassurance given.

Instead of plaster shears, some hospitals use an electric cutter for bi-valving or removing plaster. The use of the cutter requires skill, good tactile appreciation and utmost care, so that the operator will know when the cutter has cut through the plaster. As a precaution against cutting the patient's skin, it is wise to insert a cutter blade between the plaster and the patient's skin. Two people are required—one to operate the cutter, and the other to hold the child to prevent any sudden movement. Reassurance is essential because the noise of the motor may be terrifying.

After removal of the plaster, the skin should be cleaned gently and powdered with dusting powder.

The Dorsal Slab

These are plaster of Paris slabs which encircle three-quarters of the forearm. They are secured with gauze or cotton bandages wound around and completely encircling the forearm while the slab is still wet. The advantage of this application is that the plaster can be loosened easily if swelling is extensive and is likely to interfere with the circulation. This application is useful in a displacement of the distal radial epiphysis.

Batchelor Plaster of Paris

Batchelor plaster of Paris splints can be applied and used in the continuation of the treatment of congenital dislocation of the hip. Plaster of Paris is applied with the hips in full abduction and internal rotation. This position allows the femoral heads to mould as growth takes place. When the child adopts the sitting position she moves the pelvis on the femora. There is flexion and extension permitted at the hip joints. The plaster of Paris splint extends from the groin to the ankle and the legs are connected by a wooden bar, applied above the ankles.

Nursing presents few problems. The child is observed frequently to ensure that she does not remain too long in a harmful position and later she is encouraged to sit up and play without support. The child will soon show an eagerness to move herself about the floor and reach for her own toys. It is sometimes advisable to cover the plaster with some waterproof material in the region of the genitals, to avoid contamination. In very young children a suitable receptacle could be placed in position until regular habits are established.

REQUIREMENTS:

1. Pillows.
2. Table covered with a mackintosh.
3. Cotton wool.
4. Plaster of Paris bandages.
5. Wooden bar.
6. Two buckets of water.
7. X-ray plates.

POSITION OF THE CHILD. The child lies on the table with her head resting on a pillow. A warm garment may be worn over the top half of the trunk.

METHOD. The surgeon applies cotton wool over each limb from the ankle to the groin. He then manipulates the hips into the desired corrected position and with assistance applies the plaster of Paris over the wool. The wooden bar is carefully fixed in a position allowing the correction of the hips to be maintained. The plaster is then allowed to dry. When drying the back of the splint, care should be taken to protect the toes and prevent them from digging into the bed. Sandbags or a wooden rest should be used to facilitate more thorough drying and to remove pressure from the toes.

The Divaricator (Barlow's Type)

This splint may be used instead of plaster of Paris in the treatment of congenital dislocation of hips in infants up to about three months of age. It is particularly useful for nursing the child at home, since it enables the mother to change the infant's napkin, and, because of its lightness, handle the child without difficulty.

The splint is made of malleable metal and is covered with chamois leather. It is moulded to the figure of the child, fitting over the shoulders and under the thighs. The legs are held in abduction by winding the covered metal straps around the legs (Figs. 78 and 79).

While the splint is in position it is important to ensure that the parts of the malleable splint which are curled round the thighs are

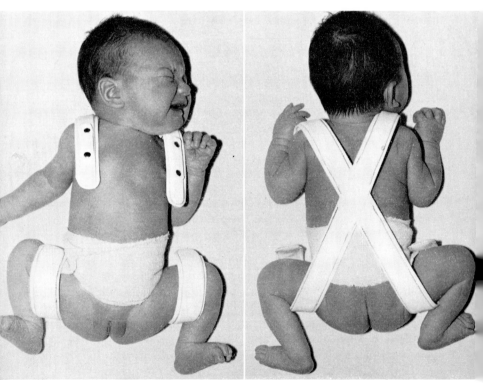

Figs. 78 & 79
Barlow's divaricator—front and back view

not too tight. Chafing may occur particularly at the top of the calf behind the knee and at the side of the neck. If vinyl covering is used the infant's skin may become sensitive to this material. This can be treated effectively with the application of zinc and castor oil cream and separating the skin from the splint by a layer of gauze.

The Divaricator (Craig's Type)

This is an adjustable splint made of plastic material with padded edges. It is used as a continuation to the Barlow type for infants over three months of age, in the treatment of congenital dislocation of hip. The napkin is placed lengthwise on the infant and held in position by the splint (Figs. 80 and 81). Napkin changes and cleaning of the area can be carried out without any difficulty.

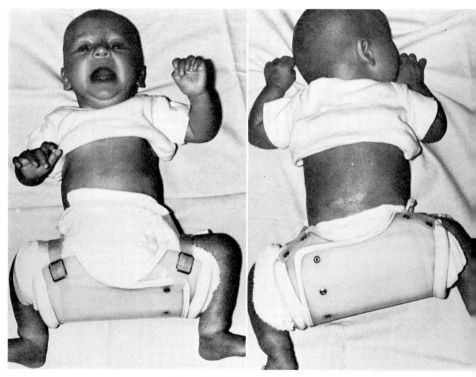

FIGS. 80 & 81
Craig's divaricator—front and back view

BIBLIOGRAPHY

Barlow, T. G. (1968). Congenital dislocation of the hip. *Nurs. Mirror*, **126**, 13.

Davies, W. T. (1959), *Aids to Orthopaedics for Nurses*. London: Baillière.

Mason Brown, J. J. (1962). *Surgery of Childhood*. London: Arnold.

Nicoll, K. B. (1963). Understanding traction. *Nurs. Times*, **59**, 1142, 1170, 1203, 1239, 1284, 1326, 1359, 1389, 1412.

Powell, M. (1968). *Orthopaedic Nursing*, 6th ed. Edinburgh: Livingstone.

CHAPTER XIX

PHYSIOTHERAPY

Miss B. G. Henderson, m.c.s.p.

I N the following chapter, I have endeavoured to explain some
physiotherapeutic procedures that a nurse may require to use
in the course of her daily routine. Simple types of procedures
are given which are readily understood and which a nurse could
carry out without the highly specialised physiotherapy training.
The need for a nurse to give physiotherapeutic treatment may
arise because of the shortage of trained physiotherapists, or when
treatment is required at unexpected times during the night.

Some more elaborate physiotherapy may be carried out by the
nurse in an emergency; e.g., postural drainage may be required
urgently for a child who has inhaled a foreign body and is admitted
at night when a physiotherapist is not available immediately.

POSTURAL DRAINAGE

Postural drainage is a procedure in which gravity is used to assist
the drainage of mucus from the lungs and encourage expectoration.
This form of treatment is usually requested for children with
bronchitis, bronchiectasis, unresolved pneumonia, and pulmonary
collapse when the acute phase is past. It may also be asked for in
the treatment of children with asthma, but here care must be
taken as the continued effort of emphasising expiration may
produce an asthmatic attack.

The postural drainage positions vary according to the area of
lung to be treated. Therefore, it is imperative that the affected
area is known before commencing treatment. The positions are
as follows:

Lower Lobes, Right and Left Lungs

1. Posterior Basal and Dorsal Bronchi. Child lies prone on
tipping pillow or bed, the apex of which is at hip level so that the

lower limbs and the trunk form an angle of 90 to 100 degrees (Figs. 82 and 83).

2. LATERAL BASAL BRONCHI. The child lies on his side with affected side uppermost. The foot of the bed is raised fourteen inches (Fig. 84).

3. ANTERIOR BASAL BRONCHI. The child lies supine; i.e., on his back, with the foot of the bed raised 14 in. (Fig. 85).

Right Mid Lobe or Left Lingula

1. The foot of the bed is raised 12 in., while the child lies on the unaffected side, midway between side lying and supine lying. This can be achieved by asking him to lie on his side, placing a pillow under his shoulder and buttock of the affected side, the child then rolling back against the pillow (Fig. 86).

In the positions for lower lobes, mid lobe and left lingula, the head must remain in the lowest possible position without a pillow.

Upper Lobes, Right and Left Lungs

1. PECTORAL OR ANTERIOR BRONCHI. Child lies supine without pillows (Fig. 87).

2. APICAL BRONCHI. Child sits upright with back supported (Fig. 88).

3. SUB-APICAL OR DORSAL BRONCHI. Child lies prone, with a pillow arranged under the shoulder of the affected side to raise that shoulder 12 in. from the bed. Figures 89 and 90 show slight difference of position for right and left upper lobes.

Each position required for the affected part is maintained for twenty to thirty minutes, thus making three or four treatments a day necessary to ensure that all parts are drained. Children under two years old are usually treated on the operator's knee, the positions being adapted to suit the size of the child. It is better to posturally drain a child immediately before a meal as the coughing can cause vomiting.

During the time the position is maintained, expiration is encouraged to increase the gaseous interchange within the lungs.

Two massage movements are employed in postural drainage. Although a description is given, they should only be used by a nurse who has been shown how to do them by the physiotherapist.

Shaking of the chest wall over the affected area is performed during expiration only. This movement is performed by placing

LOWER
LOBE

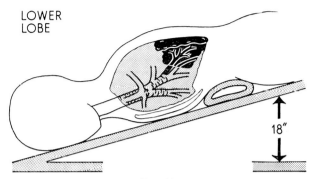

FIG. 82

Postural drainage position. Lower lobe, posterior basal bronchi.

LOWER
LOBE

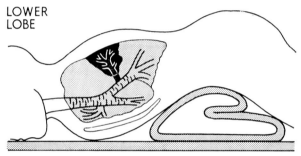

FIG. 83

Postural drainage position. Lower lobe, dorsal bronchi.

LOWER
LOBE

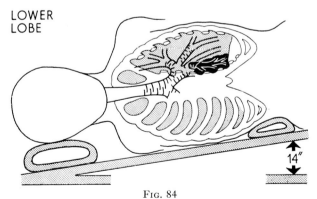

FIG. 84

Postural drainage position. Lower lobe (left), lateral basal
bronchi.

LOWER
LOBE

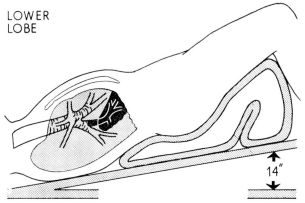

14″

FIG. 85
Postural drainage position. Lower lobe, anterior basal bronchi.

L. LINGULA

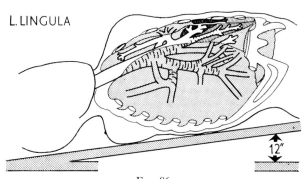

12″

FIG. 86
Postural drainage position. Left lingula.

UPPER
LOBE

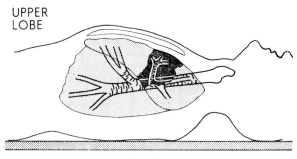

FIG. 87
Postural drainage position. Upper lobe, pectoral or anterior
bronchi.

UPPER
LOBE

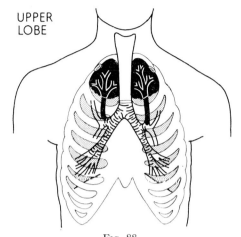

FIG. 88
Postural drainage position. Upper lobe, apical bronchi.

the palms of the hands over the area to be treated and quickly
flexing and extending the wrists but producing the slightest
possible movement. Shaking encourages deeper and fuller respirations. The movement is exhausting for the operator, who should
practise deep breathing and relaxation during its performance.

The other massage movement used during postural drainage is
clapping. This is performed by cupping the hands and giving the
part to be treated a succession of short, brisk claps. Clapping
increases cell activity within the lung and facilitates expectoration.

UPPER
LOBE

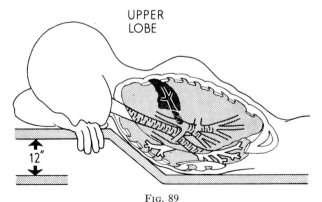

12″

FIG. 89
Postural drainage position. Upper lobe (left). sub-apical or
dorsal bronchi.

UPPER
LOBE

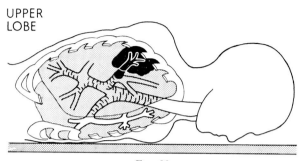

FIG. 90
Postural drainage position. Upper lobe (right), sub-apical or
dorsal bronchi.

The cupping of the hand is most important as it forms a cushion of air between the palm and the chest wall, which is necessary for the comfort of the patient.

POSTURAL DRAINAGE CAN ALSO BE REQUESTED FOR CHILDREN AFTER OPERATION. These are treated similarly to children in a medical ward, but care has to be taken not to stretch the wound; for example, you would not place a child after appendicectomy in prone lying. After thoracic or abdominal operations, the site of the wound must be supported by having the knees bent and a hand, either the patient's or the operator's, exerting gentle pressure over the wound during attempts to cough.

Children do not always understand the command 'Take a deep breath', but even a two-year-old knows how to blow. The longer they blow out, the greater inspiration they will have to make. Blowing games are used to make young children breathe deeper. There are three main types of breathing that are emphasised in treating chest conditions. These are lateral costal, diaphragmatic, and apical.

Lateral Costal Breathing is encouraged by placing the hands over the lower part of the chest wall and asking the child to push the hands out by filling themselves with air.

Diaphragmatic Breathing is more difficult to teach. Very young children are taught to make a sound like a train—'choo, choo, choo'. If enough force is put into the word, the diaphragm can be felt moving below the ziphoid process. Older children are asked to imagine they have a balloon in the triangle below the ribs so that when they breathe in, the balloon fills with air, and when they breathe out it goes flat.

Apical Breathing can be obtained by asking the child to fill his or her head with air right up to the eyebrows. This makes the child use the apical part of the lungs.

Teaching coughing to children is done by asking them to puff out air in short sharp breaths similar to the sound 'choo, choo, choo'.

When they have recovered sufficiently to get up, all children with chest conditions should be encouraged to be as active as possible.

BIBLIOGRAPHY

Nursing Times (1963). *Physiotherapy Helps Nursing.* London: Macmillan.

CHAPTER XX

RESUSCITATIVE MEASURES

Signs of respiratory obstruction; suction; ventilation; expired air resuscitation; external cardiac massage; defibrillation; drugs for cardiac arrest.

Measures which may be initiated by the nursing staff:

1. CLEARING A BLOCKED OR PARTIALLY BLOCKED AIRWAY.
2. ADMINISTRATION OF OXYGEN (Chapter XII).
3. EXPIRED AIR RESUSCITATION.
4. EXTERNAL CARDIAC MASSAGE.

Methods of resuscitation should be known to all members of the nursing staff. It is wise to have an established policy so that, in the event of an emergency, lack of knowledge does not waste vital moments in what may be a life saving measure.

Essential equipment and drugs should be an agreed part of ward policy. They should be readily available in a position known to all members of the staff.

Signs of Increasing Respiratory Embarrassment and Impending Obstruction

1. ACCESSORY BREATH SOUNDS.

(*a*) *Development of sterterous breathing* when a rattle is heard at the back of the throat. This occurs on inspiration and expiration as air is forced through accumulated secretions in the pharynx.

(*b*) *Laryngeal stridor.* This is an inspiratory stridor and occurs when obstruction is at the level of the vocal cords. The inspiration is long and drawn out in an effort to get adequate air past the obstruction.

(*c*) *Expiratory stridor.* The classical picture is that of the asthmatic when there is a forced expiratory effort in an endeavour to relieve the build up of pressure caused by spasm in the bronchioles. Partial obstruction in either bronchus will give the same picture.

2. PARADOXICAL RESPIRATION WITH INCREASED RESPIRATORY RATE. The accessory muscles of respiration are used forcefully when the main muscles of respiration, the diaphragm and the external intercostal muscles, fail to provide an adequate exchange of gases. On inspiration, there is a noticeable indraw above the manubrium sterni, the abdominal muscles are relaxed and the abdomen appears blown out. There is a forced expiration when the abdominal muscles contract, thus increasing the intra-abdominal pressure in an effort to aid in the ascent of the diaphragm.

3. INCREASED PULSE RATE will occur when some degree of anoxia is present. The heart is endeavouring to maintain the oxygen requirement of the body by circulating blood more rapidly.

4. CYANOSIS will occur gradually or rapidly depending upon the severity of the respiratory embarrassment. It is not a warning as such, but rather an indication of the degree of obstruction.

CLEARING A BLOCKED OR PARTIALLY BLOCKED AIRWAY

REQUIREMENTS:

1. Suction apparatus giving 25-38 cm. Hg, or 10-15 inches Hg vacuum.
2. Supply of sterile catheters (disposable), whistle tipped with two side holes.
3. Pressure tubing and connection.
4. Water to clear catheter.
5. Paper tissues.
6. Receptacle for disposable items.

Additional requirements when procedure is carried out using an aseptic technique; e.g., tracheal or bronchial suction:

1. Sterile glove or forceps.
2. Sterile swabs.
3. Sterile water.
4. Laryngoscope or bronchoscope.
5. Endotracheal tube of appropriate size.

Pharyngeal Suction. METHOD. The child is placed in the lateral position, or on his back with head extended (Fig. 91). If necessary, the oral cavity is cleared of debris using paper tissues. The catheter is connected, suction commenced, and the oropharynx aspirated, using gentle movements. The catheter is cleared. The pressure is occluded as the catheter is passed to the

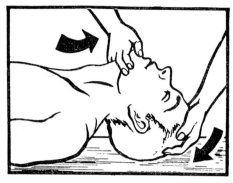

FIG. 91

posterior pharynx; it should not be passed beyond the laryngo-pharynx. The pressure is released and the catheter withdrawn gently as secretions are aspirated. The catheter is cleared and the procedure repeated. If secretions are not being obtained and no improvement is apparent, tracheal or bronchial suction will be required. Trauma to the posterior pharyngeal wall can occur when repeated suction is carried out with excessive zeal. This can cause haemorrhage, or oedema, and further embarrass respiration.

Tracheal or Bronchial Suction. This can be performed indirectly; that is, without direct vision, by a person practised in the technique; it is more usual for a laryngoscope or bronchoscope to be used. The dangers are trauma and collapse of lung through excessive use of suction without adequate ventilation of the lungs. After every third attempt to clear the airway, ventilation is necessary. As with pharyngeal suction, the catheter is inserted with the pressure occluded and suction only commenced once the catheter is in position; the catheter is gently withdrawn as soon as suction is commenced.

Equipment for Ventilation. Requirements vary depending on the age-group and the operator's preference. It is important that agreement is reached within each unit and that the equipment is in good working order and readily available.

Basic needs are:

1. Oxygen, flow meter and antistatic pressure tubing.
2. Endoscope with appropriate blades.
3. Endotracheal tubes of appropriate size.
4. Face mask, rebreathing bag and connections.

MOUTH-TO-MOUTH, MOUTH-TO-NOSE BREATHING, OR EXPIRED AIR RESUSCITATION

This method of artificial respiration has been shown to be superior to other recognised techniques of ventilation such as Schafer and Holger Nielsen. It effectively uses the expiratory muscles of the person carrying out the manoeuvre as a means of inflating the victim's lungs.

It may not be immediately obvious how expired air can be adequate to produce oxygenation but if the table below is studied, it will be seen that expired air contains between 14 and 18 per cent oxygen.

Gas	Atmospheric air %	Expired air %
Oxygen	21	14-18
Carbon Dioxide	0·04	4·5

It has been shown that the patient's oxygen saturation (normally 95 per cent saturation) will be lower than normal, but, if effective expired air resuscitation is carried out, an oxygen saturation of 80 per cent may be achieved. In addition, carbon dioxide in the patient's lungs will be effectively removed and blown off into the atmosphere. At the same time, it appears that satisfactorily low levels of carbon dioxide can be maintained for at least a half hour.

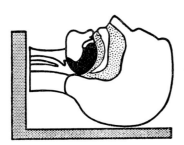 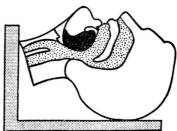

<table>
<tr><td>Fig. 92
Tongue obstructing airway with
bad position of head.</td><td>Fig. 93
Extension of head to maintain
maximum airway.</td></tr>
</table>

METHOD.

1. The patient is placed on his back.

2. The head is tilted back by extending the neck; the airway is cleared of mucus and the lower jaw supported with the right hand to keep the tongue forward (Fig. 91-93).

3. The operator's mouth is placed over the patient's mouth and with the left hand the patient's nose is pinched to prevent escape of air. In the case of the child under three years old, the operator's mouth will cover the child's mouth and nostrils (Fig. 94).

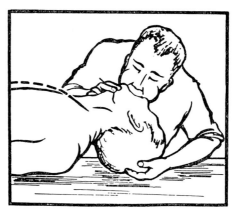

Fig. 94
Direct artificial respiration

4. Using sufficient pressure to cause the patient's chest to rise, the operator blows into the patient. If the stomach fills with air, the child is turned on to his side and pressure is applied to the epigastrium to empty the stomach of air. If regurgitation occurs along with expulsion of air, the gastric contents must be cleared before continuing. The patient is returned to the supine position and the head position is then adjusted to produce a good airway.

5. The procedure is repeated at a rate of 15 to 20 times per minute until the child is breathing adequately, or until the patient can be intubated.

6. In mouth to nose resuscitation, the right hand not only supports the lower jaw but seals the lips, and the operator blows down the nose.

The disadvantages of expired air resuscitation all lie with the person carrying out the technique. Many will find the method aesthetically repugnant, but it should be remembered that it is a life-saving technique. Infection may be a hazard in special cases; e.g., diphtheria, but these cases will be in the minority and by and large the risk of infection will be minimal.

Finally, this technique requires no apparatus, but it requires training. It is known to be better than any other first-aid method and it is available immediately at the scene of an accident, e.g. suffocation, drowning or electrocution.

The technique is most easily learned on a model such as the AMBU Manikin. Whilst this is being taught, the opportunity should be taken to learn the use of the various appliances available; e.g., *Brook airway*, and the various appliances for atmospheric air resuscitation; e.g., the *Ambu bag*, or the *Cardiff bellows*, but such appliances are not essential for effective resuscitation and furthermore, if they are not immediately available delay may occur in establishing energetic treatment.

EXTERNAL CARDIAC MASSAGE

Although it is said that brain damage is irreversible following cessation of cerebral blood flow for a period of three minutes, it should be remembered that brain damage begins to occur as soon as that organ ceases to be perfused with oxygenated blood. It should, therefore, be obvious that the person who should initiate cardiac massage is the person who first decides that cardiac arrest has occurred; this may be the nurse in training. It is important that there is some understanding of the principles involved.

ANATOMY. The heart lies within the pericardial sac. This fibroserous sac is continuous with the external coats of the great vessels superiorly and is attached inferiorly to the central tendon of the diaphragm. The heart lies, therefore, in the mediastinum, behind the body of the sternum and the cartilages of the ribs from the second to the sixth inclusive, and in front of the thoracic vertebrae.

MECHANISM. The heart is suspended within, but between the attachments of, the pericardium and cannot be displaced from side to side in the chest. Therefore, when the sternum is depressed forcibly, the heart is squeezed between the sternum and the thoracic vertebral bodies. Since the valves of the heart allow blood flow to occur in one direction, the blood in the left ventricles will be ejected into the aorta and therefore produce arterial flow.

Signs of Cardiac Arrest

1. Colour: (*a*) Skin—waxen or ash grey.
   (*b*) Mucous membrane—cyanosed or white.
2. Respiration: (*a*) Absent.
   (*b*) Apneustic.
3. Pulse—absent in a major artery such as carotid or femoral.
4. Pupils—dilated.
5. Heart sounds—absent (if a stethoscope is not immediately to hand, the ear is placed against the precardium).

METHOD.

(*a*) *Older children*

1. The child is placed on his back on a firm surface; e.g., the floor or, if it is a baby, a locker top. If the surface is soft, the massage will be ineffective and the energy will be expended on compressing bed springs or the mattress. *Note time.*

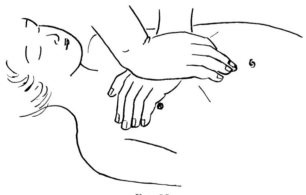

FIG. 95

External cardiac massage—the older child. Note the heel of the lower hand is placed over the lower third of the sternum.

2. The heel of one hand is placed over the lower third of the sternum and the other hand is placed on top (Fig. 95).
3. The chest wall is compressed with a thrusting motion at a rate of approximately 60-70 compressions per minute.

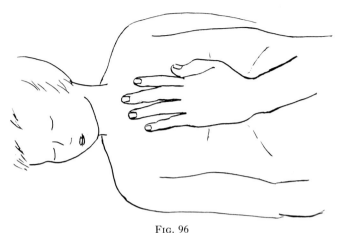

FIG. 96

External cardiac massage—the small child. Note the heel of the
hand is placed over the lower third of the sternum.

(b) Small children and infants.

4. In small children, massage may be carried out using the heel
of one hand only (Fig. 96). In newborn babies, the tips of two
fingers usually provide sufficient pressure to produce the required
effect (Fig. 97).

5. Respiration must be supported if it is not present, otherwise
external cardiac massage will be of no value. If another person is
present, expired air resuscitation may be carried out at the same

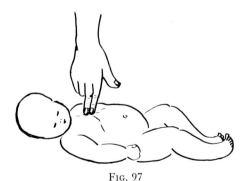

FIG. 97

External cardiac massage—newborn infant.
Note the tips of two fingers are placed on the
middle third of the sternum.

time as cardiac massage. This is best achieved with four sternal compressions, then a pause to allow the lungs to be inflated.

Signs of Effective Cardiac Massage. These signs are the reverse of the signs of cardiac arrest:

1. Improvement of colour—the lips may remain cyanosed until rubbed.
2. Palpable pulse in a major vessel—this may be difficult to determine in a small child with the vibration of massage.
3. Pupils—contracting to a smaller size. This is the most favourable of all signs as it indicates adequate perfusion of the brain.

It should be noted that no mention of drugs has been made so far. The first-aid treatment is as above and drugs are of no value until the form of cardiac arrest has been determined. The type of cardiac arrest is determined by electrocardiogram.

CARDIAC ARREST MAY OCCUR IN TWO FORMS:

1. *Asystole.*
2. *Ventricular fibrillation.*

Massage is continued in both states. Sodium bicarbonate is given to counter the metabolic acidosis associated with hypoxia of arrest, starting with 1 mEq per Kg.

ASYSTOLE. In the case of asystole, cardiac massage is continued for at least 10 minutes before further measures are contemplated. During this time, the heart may begin to beat unaided when it will be possible to stop massage.

If the contractions are weak, then it may be necessary for adrenaline to be injected into the chamber of the left ventricle. If the blood pressure remains low (below 80 mm. Hg) it will be necessary to give a slow noradrenaline intravenous infusion. If the heart remains in asystole, the muscle tone of the heart will be improved by injecting calcium chloride 10 per cent solution (0·1 ml./Kg.) intravenously or directly into the heart. If asystole persists, massage is continued until the heart fails to fill in diastole or until signs of permanent brain damage are present. How long one should persist with cardiac massage must be left to the doctor in charge to decide.

Defibrillation

VENTRICULAR FIBRILLATION. The treatment of ventricular fibrillation is by electrical defibrillation. Defibrillators may be of two types:

1. Internal defibrillators act by using a voltage below 250 volts and many are of variable voltage; e.g., 100 volts and 220 volts. The current is allowed to pass for 0·1 second by the apparatus.

2. External defibrillators act by using voltages between 500 volts and 1,000 volts. They normally allow a choice of several voltages from the one apparatus. With the voltage being so high, it is wise to ensure that no part of the person carrying out the procedure, or any assistant, is in contact with the patient during defibrillation. If one single electrical impulse does not convert the ventricular rhythm to normal rhythm or asystole, then up to three shocks in rapid succession may prove successful.

External defibrillators are the apparatus of choice when external massage has been carried out. Both types of defibrillator may cause burns of the patient, and particularly so if insufficient care is taken in providing the correct saline pad or pads.

If the heart returns to normal rhythm following defibrillation, then the treatment is as described where the heart returns to normal rhythm following massage alone. If the heart goes to asystole, then the treatment is as described for asystole.

Complications

1. Fractured ribs—this is not common in childhood.
2. Ruptured liver—the liver may be large and tense before carrying out massage, and careless, rough technique may damage it.
3. Marrow embolism—has been reported

Contra-indications to External Massage.

Where the pericardial sac has been opened or removed at surgery, the heart will merely undergo a pendulum motion in the chest and the open method of massage is the one of choice.

Drugs to be Kept on Cardiac Arrest Trolley

1. Sodium bicarbonate 8·4 per cent solution (1 mEq/ml.)— corrects metabolic acidosis.

2. Adrenaline 1:1000 solution—cardiac stimulant.
3. Noradrenaline—vaso-constrictor, raises blood pressure.
4. Calcium chloride 10 per cent solution—cardiac stimulant.
5. Hydrocortisone sodium succinate—general stimulant.
6. Atropine sulphate—inhibitor of vagal nerve impulses.
7. Isoprenaline—cardiac stimulant.

It should be noted that Kouwenhoven et al. (1960) reported a series in which the age-group of 20 patients varied from 2 months to 80 years. In 13 of these cases, artificial ventilation was carried out simultaneously and the duration of massage ranged from one minute to sixty-five minutes. The hearts of three of the patients were in ventricular fibrillation and they were defibrillated by a closed chest defibrillator. All twenty cases were resuscitated and, at the time of publication, fourteen were alive with intellect unimpaired.

The real value of external cardiac massage lies in the fact that it may be used wherever the emergency arises either at the roadside or bedside.

BIBLIOGRAPHY

Feldman, S. & Ellis, H. (1967). *Principles of Resuscitation.* Oxford: Blackwell.

Kouwenhoven, W. B., Jude, J. R. & Knicker-bocker, G. G. (1960). Closed chest cardiac massage. *J. Am. med. Ass.*, **173**, 1064.

Smith & Nephew, Ltd. (1962). *Direct Artificial Respiration* (Information Handbook).

APPENDIX A

SOME DISINFECTANTS IN CURRENT USE

A few disinfectants in current use have been listed. They by no means cover the variety available. It is important to study available literature to ensure that the disinfectant and its strength are suitable for the purpose.

Purpose	Disinfectant	Strength	Remarks
1. *Skin disinfection*	pHisohex Sterzac		Hexachloro- phane deter- gent washing creams
	Betadine scrub	$\frac{3}{4}\%$ available iodine	Povidone-iodine cream
	Chlorhexidine tincture	0·5% in 70% alcohol	Skin preparation
	Savlon	1 in 30 in 70% alcohol	Skin preparation
	Iodine	1% in 70% alcohol	Skin preparation
2. *Wounds*	Chlorhexidine	1 in 2,000	
	Savlon	1 in 100	1 in 30 for gross- ly contamin- ated wounds
3. *Emergency disinfec-* *tion of instruments*	Chlorhexidine tincture	0·5% in 70% alcohol	Immerse for 2 min.
	Savlon	1 in 30 in 70% alcohol	Immerse for 2 min.
	Chlorhexidine gluconate	0·5% in 70% alcohol	Immerse for 2 min.
4. *Napkin rinse to* *prevent napkin der-* *matitis*	Benzalkonium chloride	1 in 80	Soak for 30 min. after final rinse
	Chlorhexidine	1 in 10,000	Used as final rinse
5. *Linen, contamina-* *ted, typhoid or* *paratyphoid*	Sudol	1 in 80	Soak for 1 hour.

Purpose	Disinfectant	Strength	Remarks
6. General purposes: surface disinfection, trolleys etc.	Benzalkonium chloride	1 in 40	Wash liberally and allow to dry.
	Chlorhexidine	1 in 5,000	
	Savlon	1 in 200	
	Cetrimide 1% stock B.P.	1 in 2	
7. Respirators and incubators	Chlorhexidine gluconate in distilled water	1 in 5,000	Use in humidifier.
	Sudol	1 in 120	Wash liberally and allow to dry.
8. Thermometers	Isopropanol	70%	2 min.
	Savlon	1 in 30 in 70% alcohol	2 min.
9. Baths	Savlon	1 in 200	All disinfectants: Wash liberally and rinse after 5 min.
	Sudol	1 in 20	
	Benzalkonium chloride	1 in 10	
	Chloros	1 in 80	
10. Plastic mugs	Milton	1 in 80	One hour
	Benzalkonium chloride	1 in 40	One hour
11. Baby bottles and teats	Milton	1 in 80	Immerse for 1½ hours. Change every 24 hours
12. Faeces—typhoid or paratyphoid	Sudol	1 in 80	Cover for one hour before emptying.

BRITISH PHARMACOPOEIA NAME AND PROPRIETARY
EQUIVALENT

Chlorhexidine: 'Hibitane'
Cetrimide B.P.:   'Cetavlon'
Benzalkonium Chloride: 'Roccal'
Chlorhexidine with Cetrimide B.P.:   'Savlon'

APPENDIX B

THE RESTRAINER SLEEVE

The restrainer sleeve (Fig. 42) can be readily made from linen. Wooden spatulae are inserted into five slots in the sleeve. The sleeve from A to B is double material.

Measurements	Infant size	Toddler size
A–B	7 in.	8 in.
C–D	9 in.	10 in.
E–A	12 in.	15 in.
Circumference at B	$5\frac{1}{2}$ in.	$6\frac{1}{2}$ in.
Circumference at A	8 in.	9 in.

Note: Point A is on the shoulder and tapes E tie under the opposite arm.

INDEX

Tracheostomy, 168
cleansing of airway, 171
position of child, 170
Traction fixed, 302
gallows, 305
long axis, 300
sliding, 304
weight and pulley, 303
Trauma, emotional, 2
Trypsin, in duodenal juice, 275
in faeces, 284
Tryptic activity, 275
Turning frame, 316

Underwater seal drainage, 176
dangers in, 179
measurement of drainage, 179
position of bottle, 178
physiological principle in, 176
removal of catheter, 180
suction in, 178
Undine, 145
Urea clearance test, 223
Urea concentration test, 223
Urine, clean catch, 211
collecting bag, 209
collection of specimen, 206
mid-stream specimen, 211
preparation of test tube, 207
retention of, 217
single specimen, female infant, 211
single specimen, male infant, 207
24-hour collection, female, 213
24-hour collection, male, 211
Urine tests, for bilirubin, 293
for blood, 292
for chlorides, 287
for ketone bodies, 291
for phenylketonuria, 294
for protein, 288
for pus, 294
for sugar, 290
general examination, 286
reaction of, 287

Venepuncture, 228
for administration of fluids, 232
Venesection, for administration of
fluids, 233
Ventilation, 35
Ventilation, positive pressure, 172
mechanical, 174
Ventricular puncture, 137
Ventriculography, 259, 260
Vertigo, syringing of ear, 149
Visiting of children, 2, 9, 11
Visitors, 34
Vital signs, convulsions, 25
head injury, 24
Voiding cystogram, 264

Ward dressings, 71
methods of, 74
preparation of child for, 71
principles of technique, 72
specific techniques, 75
Airstrip ward dressing, 81
corset dressing, 80
finger dressing, 85
removal of sutures, 75
shortening of peritoneal tube, 84
Ward infection, 29
dangers of, 30
in infants, 31
observation and reporting, 43
prevention and spread of, 32
sources of, 29
Staphylococcus in, 30, 31
visitors in, 34
Water intoxication, 202
Watershed dressing, 82
Weight and pulley traction, 304
Weights and measures, 125
approximate equivalents, 127
conversion tables, 129, 130, 132
Imperial system, 126
metric system, 126
Wound healing, 81

PRINTED IN GREAT BRITAIN BY ROBERT CUNNINGHAM AND SONS LTD., ALVA